T0230498

Global Maternal and Child Health

Medical, Anthropological, and Public Health Perspectives

Series Editor
David A. Schwartz, Atlanta, GA, USA

Global Maternal and Child Health: Medical, Anthropological, and Public Health Perspectives is a series of books that will provide the most comprehensive and current sources of information on a wide range of topics related to global maternal and child health, written by a collection of international experts.

The health of pregnant women and their children are among the most significant public health, medical, and humanitarian problems in the world today. Because in developing countries many people are poor, and young women are the poorest of the poor, persistent poverty exacerbates maternal and child morbidity and mortality and gender-based challenges to such basic human rights as education and access to health care and reproductive choices. Women and their children remain the most vulnerable members of our society and, as a result, are the most impacted individuals by many of the threats that are prevalent, and, in some cases, increasing throughout the world. These include emerging and re-emerging infectious diseases, natural and man-made disasters, armed conflict, religious and political turmoil, relocation as refugees, malnutrition, and, in some cases, starvation. The status of indigenous women and children is especially precarious in many regions because of ethnic, cultural, and language differences, resulting in stigmatization, poor obstetrical and neonatal outcomes, limitations of women's reproductive rights, and lack of access to family planning and education that restrict choices regarding their own futures. Because of the inaccessibility of women to contraception and elective pregnancy termination, unsafe abortion continues to result in maternal deaths, morbidity, and reproductive complications. Unfortunately, maternal deaths remain at unacceptably high levels in the majority of developing countries, as well as in some developed ones. Stillbirths and premature deliveries result in millions of deaths annually. Gender inequality persists globally as evidenced by the occurrence of female genital mutilation, obstetrical violence, human trafficking, and other forms of sexual discrimination directed at women. Many children are routinely exposed to physical, sexual, and psychological violence. Childhood and teen marriages remain at undesirably high levels in many developing countries.

Global Maternal and Child Health: Medical, Anthropological, and Public Health Perspectives is unique in combining the opinions and expertise of public health specialists, physicians, anthropologists and social scientists, epidemiologists, nurses, midwives, and representatives of governmental and non governmental agencies to. comprehensively explore the increasing challenges and potential solutions to global maternal and child health issues.

Barbara A. Anderson • Lisa R. Roberts
Editors

Maternal Health and American Cultural Values

Beyond the Social Determinants

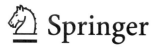 Springer

Editors
Barbara A. Anderson ⓘ
Frontier Nursing University
Versailles, KY, USA

Lisa R. Roberts ⓘ
Loma Linda University
Loma Linda, CA, USA

ISSN 2522-8382   ISSN 2522-8390   (electronic)
Global Maternal and Child Health
ISBN 978-3-031-23971-7   ISBN 978-3-031-23969-4   (eBook)
https://doi.org/10.1007/978-3-031-23969-4

© The Editor(s) (if applicable) and The Author(s), under exclusive license to Springer Nature Switzerland AG 2023
This work is subject to copyright. All rights are solely and exclusively licensed by the Publisher, whether the whole or part of the material is concerned, specifically the rights of translation, reprinting, reuse of illustrations, recitation, broadcasting, reproduction on microfilms or in any other physical way, and transmission or information storage and retrieval, electronic adaptation, computer software, or by similar or dissimilar methodology now known or hereafter developed.
The use of general descriptive names, registered names, trademarks, service marks, etc. in this publication does not imply, even in the absence of a specific statement, that such names are exempt from the relevant protective laws and regulations and therefore free for general use.
The publisher, the authors, and the editors are safe to assume that the advice and information in this book are believed to be true and accurate at the date of publication. Neither the publisher nor the authors or the editors give a warranty, expressed or implied, with respect to the material contained herein or for any errors or omissions that may have been made. The publisher remains neutral with regard to jurisdictional claims in published maps and institutional affiliations.

This Springer imprint is published by the registered company Springer Nature Switzerland AG
The registered company address is: Gewerbestrasse 11, 6330 Cham, Switzerland

We dedicate this book to all that is positive in American cultural values.

*At their best, they have sustained our nation and supported the health of **all** our mothers.*

Series Editorial Advisory Board

- **Severine Caluwaerts, M.D.,** Médecins Sans Frontières/Doctors Without Borders, Operational Centre, Brussels; and Obstetrician-Gynecologist, Institute for Tropical Medicine, Antwerp, Belgium
- **Kim Gutschow, Ph.D.,** Lecturer, Departments of Anthropology and Religion, Williams College, Williamstown, MA, USA
- **Morgan Hoke, Ph.D.,** Assistant Professor of Anthropology, University of Pennsylvania, Philadelphia, PA, USA
- **Regan Marsh, M.D., M.P.H.,** Attending Physician, Brigham and Women's Hospital; Instructor, Department of Emergency Medicine, Harvard Medical School; Affiliate Faculty, Division of Global Health Equity, Department of Medicine, Harvard Medical School; and Partners in Health, Boston, MA, USA
- **Joia Stapleton Mukherjee, M.D.,** Associate Professor of Medicine; Associate Professor of Global Health and Social Medicine, Department of Global Health & Social Medicine, Harvard University School of Medicine; and Partners in Health, Boston, MA, USA
- **Adrienne E. Strong, Ph.D.,** Assistant Professor of Anthropology, Department of Anthropology, University of Florida, Gainesville, FL, USA
- **Deborah A. Thomas, Ph.D.,** R. Jean Brownlee Term Professor of Anthropology, Interim Director, Gender, Sexuality and Women's Studies, University of Pennsylvania, Philadelphia, PA, USA; and Editor-in-Chief, American Anthropologist
- **Claudia Valeggia, Ph.D.,** Professor of Anthropology (Biological Anthropology), Department of Anthropology, Yale University, New Haven, CT, USA
- **Nynke van der Broek, Ph.D., F.R.C.O.G., D.T.M. & H.,** Head of the Centre for Maternal and Newborn Health, Professor of Maternal and Newborn Health, Honorary Consultant Obstetrician and Gynaecologist, Liverpool School of Tropical Medicine, Liverpool, UK

Preface

The health of mothers in America is among the best and worst in the world. Maternal health outcomes in our nation rank the lowest among developed nations and lower than many transitional nations. How can this be? What are the forces driving these outcomes in this wealthy nation? The national conversation points to adverse social determinants of health among so many of our mothers, e.g., poverty, limited access to health care, poor health literacy, and violence. Yet, the paradox of the healthy immigrant, excellent outcomes among immigrant mothers in the first generation facing these very challenges, remains unexplained. Can we explain away our poor maternal health outcomes by these adverse determinants of health or are there more fundamental factors at play?

America is grounded in solid and recognizable cultural values, among the most prominent being individualism, personal control, action orientation, practicality, and self-reliance. The globally recognized "can-do" attitude of Americans is reflected in action orientation and practicality. The individualism in American society is noted around the world, admired, and lamented. High cultural expectations for self-control and self-reliance frame the behavior of the American people, often disappoint us, and drive us to isolation. Our historical values can build us up or tear us down. As a nation, these values drive our healthcare decisions, policies and programs, for better and for worse. They are key to understanding *why* we have so many American mothers dying or having poor health outcomes.

This book takes a hard look at the responsibility of the nation to ask the question *why—why such poor outcomes, why pervasive adverse determinants of health?* It looks beyond these factors to an exploration of how these cultural values drive decisions by individuals, communities, and national policy and planning. With an interdisciplinary approach, the editors and contributors examine values-based decision-making among our most vulnerable mothers—those who struggle with drug addiction, incarceration, mental illness, autonomy in reproductive choice, racism. The authors propose that understanding and acknowledging the role of our American cultural values in decision-making at all levels is a powerful tool for leveraging solutions to the crisis in maternal health in America.

Part I examines the juxtaposition of maternal health, cultural values, and the social determinants of health. Part II explores the lived experiences of American mothers from a number of vantage points. Part III describes a divided nation and how it affects our mothers. Part IV delves in to the influences in our communities as they affect maternal health. Part V challenges us to look into our cultural mirror and consider the factors that enhance and undermine the health of our mothers.

This work has wide applicability for use by scholars, students, and citizens committed to using all that is good in our nation for the good of all of our people. It encourages us not to shy away from that side of our historical values that need to be exposed to the light of day and to speak truth to power. It encourages us to be the best that we, as a nation, can be.

Versailles, KY, USA   Barbara A. Anderson
Loma Linda, CA, USA   Lisa R. Roberts
September 24, 2022

Acknowledgments

We would like to acknowledge our series editor, David A. Schwartz, *Global Maternal and Child Health: Medical, Anthropological, and Public Health Perspectives*. Thank you, David, for your openness to our book topic, your valuable suggestions, and for being so approachable. We are also grateful to always-available Springer editor, Janet Kim, and Project coordinator, Olivia Ramya Chitranjan. We were honored to work with our team of authors and reviewers who shared not only their content expertise and their knowledge of the nation's public health goals but also their deep understanding of cultural values that drive decisions, positively and negatively, at all levels in our nation.

We would like to acknowledge the following persons who shared their expertise: Martha Hoffman Goedert, PhD, Clinical Professor, University of Nebraska; Nikia Grayson, DNP, Director of Clinical Services, CHOICES Memphis Center for Reproductive Health, Memphis, TN; Elise Pletnikoff, MD, Healthcare Provider, Indian Health Service, Kodiak, AK; Ann V. Millard, PhD, Associate Professor Emerita, Texas A&M University, McAllen, TX; Carolyn Sufrin, MD-PhD, Associate Professor, John Hopkins University; Heather S. Swanson, DNP, Associate Professor, Mount Marty University; Suzan Ulrich, DrPH, Program Director, George Washington University. Finally, we are grateful for the American culture that allows openness of discussion, and for those who have shown us the best side of American cultural values.

About the Book

Many women of childbearing age in the USA have poor health outcomes. The social, economic, and environmental milieu are influential. These "social determinants of health" are markers. Yet, they do not explain, at a deeper cultural level, *why* the mortality and morbidity among many American mothers are so much higher compared with other high-income and many middle-income nations.

Using an interdisciplinary, critical analysis approach, this book examines how patterns of decision-making, grounded in core American cultural values, have profoundly influenced the lived experiences and health outcomes of mothers. Part I examines the links among core cultural values, policy decisions, social conditions, and maternal health outcomes. Part II explores the lived experience of American mothers, while Part III analyzes the impact of a highly divisive nation on this experience. Part IV discusses how society shapes social determinants of health for motherhood. Part V proposes that American cultural values frame an explanatory model for decision-making with both positive and negative impacts on maternal health in America. The book is a descriptive analysis offering a framework for leverage of solutions based upon cultural values.

Contents

Contributors

Barbara A. Anderson, DrPH, Frontier Nursing University, Versailles, KY, USA

Eugene N. Anderson, PhD, University of California, Riverside, CA, USA

Cheryl Tatano Beck, DNSc, University of Connecticut, Storrs, CA, USA

Lana J. Bernat, DNP, U.S. Army Nurse Corps, HQDA OTSG, Watertown, NY, USA

Denae L. Bradley, PhD ©, Robert Wood Johnson Health Policy Research Scholar, Howard University, Hyattsville, MD, USA

Mary de Chesnay, PhD, Kennesaw State University, Kennesaw, GA, USA

Jennifer W. Foster, PhD, Emory University, Atlanta, GA, USA

Joan MacEachen, MD-MPH, Healthcare Provider, Durango, CO, USA

Linda R. McDaniel, DNP, CNM, Healthcare Provider, WellStar Medical Group Cobb Gynecologists, Austell, GA, USA

Lisa R. Roberts, DrPH, Loma Linda University, Loma Linda, CA, USA

Rachel S. Simmons, PhD, WHNP, Healthcare Provider, Southwest Orlando Family Medicine, Orlando, FL, USA

About the Editors

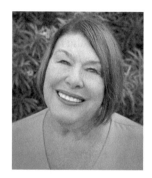

Barbara A. Anderson, DrPH, CNM, FACNM, FAAN is professor emerita and a founding director of the Doctor of Nursing Practice at Frontier Nursing University, Lexington, Kentucky. She formerly served as administrative dean at Seattle University College of Nursing, Seattle, Washington, and faculty at Loma Linda University School of Public Health, Loma Linda, California. Promoting and enabling the health of mothers is her lifelong passion and she has deep experience in the USA and globally in public health, nurse-midwifery, and university administration and education. She was lead editor of *The Maternal Health Crisis in America: Nursing Implications for Advocacy and Practice* (2019)—an American Journal of Nursing (AJN) first-place award winner and lead editor of *Best Practices in Midwifery: Using the Evidence to Implement Change* (2013, 2017), also first-place AJN award winner. She co-edited four editions of *Caring for the Vulnerable: Perspectives in Nursing Theory, Research, and Practice* (2008, 2012, 2016, 2019) and co-authored a four-volume series on genocide, *Warning Signs of Genocide* (2013-2023), based upon genocidal experiences with refugees. She currently serves on the editorial board of the *International Journal of Childbirth;* the community advisory board of an NIH-funded childhood obesity study among low-income Hispanic mothers, University of California at Riverside, School of Medicine; and on the national team for the Accreditation Commission for Midwifery Education. She received the National League of Nursing Mary Adelaide Nutting Award for Outstanding Teaching (2019) and the American Association of Birth Centers Media Award (2018). She has been on teams at Health and Human Services Office of Minority Health examining refugee health and cultural competency in maternal health care.

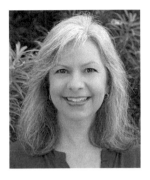

Lisa R. Roberts, Dr.PH, FNP-BC, FAANP, FAAN is professor and research director, School of Nursing, with secondary appointment in the School of Behavioral Health and a faculty scholar in the Institute for Health Policy and Leadership and the Center for Bioethics, Loma Linda University, Loma Linda, California. She maintains a full teaching load with graduate students and grant-procurement as research director. She has broad domestic and global experience in maternal health, perinatal grief, and vulnerable populations. Her research has focused on maternal vulnerability and perinatal grief. Also currently in clinical practice as a Nurse Practitioner, she has worked with multiple cultural groups in rural and urban settings in the USA and globally. She served as a consultant for Health and Human Services Office of Minority Health in the development of *Cultural competency in maternal health care* educational modules for healthcare professionals, and as a panel member for a seminar titled, *Why are Black mothers and babies in a life-or-death crisis? A lesson on the disparities in maternal and infant mortality*. In 2022 she completed a Fulbright Faculty award as a visiting scholar at Christian Medical College, Vellore, India. She is coeditor of *The Maternal Health Crisis in America: Nursing Implications for Advocacy and Practice* (2019), coeditor of *Midwifery for Nurses in India* (2018), and an author on role transition among immigrant women in *Caring for the Vulnerable: Perspectives in Nursing Theory, Practice, and Research*, 4th Ed. (2015).

List of Abbreviations and Acronyms

ACE	Adverse Childhood Events
AI/AN	American Indian and Alaskan Native
ANA	American Nurses Association
ART	Assisted Reproductive Technology
BMMA	Black Mamas Matter Alliance
CAPTA	Child Abuse Prevention and Treatment
CDC	Centers for Disease Control and Prevention
CIA	Central Intelligence Agency
CMMS	Centers for Medicare and Medicaid Services
CNM	Certified Nurse Midwife
CPS	Child Protective Services
DACA	Deferred Action on Childhood Arrivals
DNP	Doctor of Nursing Practice
DOD	Department of Defense
ECAT	Elemental Carbon Attributable to Traffic
EPA	Environmental Protection Agency
EPA	Equal Pay Act
FDA	Food and Drug Administration
FMLA	Family Medical Leave Act
HBCU	Historically Black Colleges and Universities
HIS	Indian Health Service
HMO	Health Maintenance Organization
ICFJ	International Center for Journalists
ICU	Intensive Care Unit
IPV	Intimate Partner Violence
IVF	In Vitro Fertilization
LCT	Life Course Theory
LGBTQ+	Lesbian, Gay, Bisexual, Transgender, Queer/Questioning, others
MD	Medical Doctor
MHS	Military Health System
MMR	Maternal Mortality Rate

MWR	Morale, Welfare, and Recreation Program
NAS	Neonatal Abstinence Syndrome
NICU	Neonatal Intensive Care Unit
NPIC	National Perinatal Information Center
NRA	National Rifle Association
PM	Particulate Matter
PPO	Preferred Provider Organization
PRAMS	Pregnancy Risk Assessment Monitoring System
PTSD	Posttraumatic Stress Disorder
RGV	Rio Grande Valley
RMC	Respectful Maternity Care
SDoH	Social Determinants of Health
SMP	Social Media Platforms
TTHM	Trihalomethane
UN	United Nations
UNESCO	United Nations Educational, Scientific, and Cultural Organization
UNHCR	United High Commission on Refugees
USA	United States of America
USDHHS	United States Department of Health and Human Services
WHO	World Health Organization
WIC	Special Supplemental Nutrition Program for Women, Infants, and Children

List of Boxes

Part I
Maternal Health, American Cultural Values, and the Social Determinants of Health

Chapter 1
The Health of American Mothers in the Context of Cultural Values

Barbara A. Anderson and Lisa R. Roberts

1.1 The Current State of Maternal Health in the USA

As American as motherhood and apple pie is a common expression in the United States of America (USA) to signify those customs and beliefs that are widely shared and fundamental to the culture. The expression speaks to the importance and reverence for mothers in the culture. However, many mothers in the USA face a number of high-risk situations. Overall maternal health in the USA does not compare favorably to other high-resource nations. Maternal mortality, morbidity, and near misses in the USA are the highest among high-income nations and comparable to many middle-income nations (Davis et al., 2019; Larroca et al., 2020; Tikkanen et al., 2020; Weil & Reichert, 2021; World Health Organization [WHO], 2019). The 2019 overall maternal mortality rate (MMR) of 21 per 100,000 live births continued the rising trend over the past three decades (Hoyert, 2021; Mehta et al., 2021).

B. A. Anderson (✉)
Frontier Nursing University, Versailles, KY, USA

L. R. Roberts
Loma Linda University, Loma Linda, CA, USA

© The Author(s), under exclusive license to Springer Nature Switzerland AG 2023
B. A. Anderson, L. R. Roberts (eds.), *Maternal Health and American Cultural Values*,
Global Maternal and Child Health, https://doi.org/10.1007/978-3-031-23969-4_1

Box 1.1 Trends in Pregnancy-Related Mortality in the United States

Trends in pregnancy-related mortality in the United States: 1987-2017

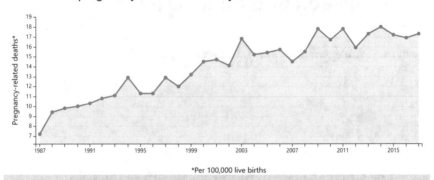

*Per 100,000 live births

(Centers for Disease Control and Prevention, 2020)

The USA ranks 55th among 184 nations in MMR despite significantly higher healthcare spending on maternity care (Central Intelligence Agency, 2021). Some low-income and a number of middle-income countries have maternal health metrics on par with the USA (WHO, 2019). Globally, maternal mortality has decreased substantially with implementation of the United Nations (UN) development goals. However, the USA has neither adopted nor implemented these proven strategies (MacDorman & Declercq, 2018). WHO has determined that the USA and the Dominican Republic are the only two nations with a true increase in MMR between 2000 and 2017 (WHO, 2019). The USA has not met the national goals for most maternal health indicators targeted in the *Healthy People 2020* document, and only baseline data is available for maternal mortality (National Center for Health Statistics, 2021).

Though maternal mortality rates, morbidity estimates, and near misses vary in how they are measured from state to state, the extant literature consistently documents high rates on average. Furthermore, hidden by the national average, these rates vary considerably between groups of various race or ethnicity. Persistently higher MMR among Black mothers is an indication of health disparities, as their MMR is 3.5 times higher than among Hispanic mothers, and 2.5 times higher than among White mothers (Amankwaa et al., 2018; Hoyert, 2021). American Indian/Alaska Native mothers have almost as high an MMR as Black mothers (United Health Foundation, 2021).

The high MMR in the USA has been attributed to high rates of obesity and lifestyle related diseases (including cardiovascular disease), advanced maternal age, and high intervention rates, impeding physiological birth (Goncalves et al., 2020; Mehta et al., 2021). Approximately two-thirds of the maternal deaths in the USA could be prevented (Davis et al., 2019). Preventable maternal mortality, morbidity, and near misses are related to contributing factors such as low health literacy, poor preconception health, delayed or ineffective treatment due to missed warning signs, and complex, fragmented healthcare and surveillance systems (Petersen et al., 2021). Maternal health remains an overlooked health crisis in the USA. The general public is often unaware of the issue. Likewise, awareness is not high among public health and healthcare providers who are not directly involved with maternal care.

1.2 Social and Environmental Conditions Affecting Maternal Health

1.2.1 The Social Determinants of Health

Social and environmental conditions influence health outcomes. The framework of the Social Determinants of Health (Healthy People 2030) provides guidance on five key domains and well referenced literature on contributing conditions.

Box 1.2 Social Determinants of Health

Domain	Elements
Economic stability	Employment/underemployment/unemployment rate (job benefits) Food insecurity (due to lack of money and other resources) Housing instability (due to cost burden of $\geq 30\%$–50% of income) Poverty (causing increased risk for disease and death)
Education access and quality	Early childhood development and education (first five years) High school graduation (standard requirement for most jobs) Enrollment in higher education (additional employment options) Language and literacy (limited oral/written English proficiency in the USA)
Health care access and quality	Access to health services (health insurance coverage, transportation and language barriers, availability of health resources) Access to primary care (as usual source of care) Health literacy (personal and organizational health literacy)
Neighborhood and built environment	Access to healthy foods (distance to supermarket) Crime and violence (experience and/or exposure) Environmental conditions (air pollution, water quality, extreme heat) Quality of housing (home safety, space per individual, maintenance)
Social and community context	Civic participation (voting, volunteering, building social capital) Discrimination (unfair socially structured action/stressor with a negative physiological effect) Incarceration rate and recidivism rate (affecting individual and family health) Social cohesion (strength of relationships and solidarity among community members)

(Healthy People 2030)

1.2.2 The Social Determinants of Maternal Health

Maternal health can be impacted by each or all of the five domains in the social determinants of health (SDoH). For example, a pregnant woman with limited education and income may experience food insecurity due to living in a neighborhood that lacks access to affordable, healthy foods. Her housing may be substandard, exposure to community violence is common, and social discrimination is high. Further, she may lack transportation to obtain basic primary healthcare services. This scenario describes social risks to her health in terms of *who, what, when, where*, and *how much*. What the SDoH do not answer is **why**, in a resource-rich environment like the USA, this pregnant woman experiences these disparities. The SDoH are not the cause of persistent poor maternal health outcomes among many women in the USA. Rather, they are the social markers of a milieu in a high resource nation that does not prioritize maternal health for all mothers and may support decisions that undermine maternal health.

Maternal health is not a priority policy agenda despite repeated calls for action (Koblinsky et al., 2012; Koblinsky et al., 2016; Mehta et al., 2021). While some historical patterns of policy and legislation have been supportive, there are other agendas that have undermined maternal health in the USA (Brunson & Suh, 2020; Kenner, et al. 2018; Thompson-Dudiak, 2021; Villines, 2019). Policies, legislation, and community action are grounded in decisions that reflect what matters, what is most important, and what is critical to society (Kelley, 2020). These decisions reflect the cultural values of a society.

1.3 Cultural Values and Maternal Health Outcomes

Cultural values are the principles that guide collective behavior and commonly held convictions and beliefs. They are transmitted within a society by parents and peers as well as politicians, religious leaders, teachers, law enforcement and others. While many cultures around the world hold similar values, they are defined, modified, and contextualized within an identified culture (Alemán & Woods, 2016). Cultural values, translated into decisions and actions, may enhance or undermine the health outcomes of a population, including that of childbearing women (National Research Council and the Institute of Medicine, 2013; United Nations, 2019; United Nations Human Rights Council, 2018).

1.3.1 American Cultural Values

American cultural values lie behind almost every structure and institution in the USA, having been enshrined by the Founding Fathers in the Constitution of the nation. These values were immortalized by Benjamin Franklin in *Poor Richard's*

Almanack and other writings (2013, orig 1732) and his *Autobiography* (Franklin 1949, 1961). The French visitor to the USA, Alexis de Tocqueville, penned rich historical detail on Franklin's description of American values (de Tocqueville 2003, orig. 1835, 1840).

American cultural values are clearly on the national radar when any complicated decision is made in the USA, as evidenced by recent discussions on abortion in the Supreme Court. They shade every decision, even if not explicit, including COVID-19 vaccination uptake and refusal. Even if an individual American does not espouse all of these values, broad cultural exposure is inescapable. Any value that is commonly held will be praised far beyond its actual presence, if only to encourage those with less commitment to comply. These values, translated into decisions and actions, have great potential for enhancing or undermining the health of the population, including maternal health. Viewed through this perspective raises the question: ***why*** does the USA have such poor maternal outcomes? This work explores American cultural values that influence decisions about resource distribution for maternal health and the impact of the SDoH as markers of maternal life course in the USA.

A literature search revealed five key American values with strong scholarship. Subsequent Delphi technique with social scientists, public health professionals, and healthcare providers ($n = 12$) resulted in independent and high agreement on their prevalence as key American values and their potential for impact on maternal health. These cultural values are:

- Personal control.
- Individualism.
- Action-orientation.
- Practicality.
- Self-reliance.

1.3.2   Personal Control

Personal control is highly valued in the American culture. It implies the ability to control one's self and one's environment. It shapes an individual's belief about the degree to which one can influence events, both positive and negative. It can affect how one perceives the fairness of life's contingencies (Lerner, 1980). The opposite is a sense of personal powerlessness and fatalism. Julian Rotter (1966) developed the concept of *locus of control* which speaks to an individual's understanding of personal control. Albert Bandura describes this value in describing *self-efficacy* (1982, 1997) and *social cognitive theory* (1986, 1989). William Glasser's *control theory* centers on how we control our lives (1985). More recent scholarship describes life course trajectories, health behavior, and resiliency through the cultural lens of personal control (Baumeister, 2015; Cusimano & Goodwin, 2020; Galla & Duckworth, 2015; Infurna et al., 2013; Mirowsky & Ross, 2007; Ryon & Gleason, 2018).

American mothers are immersed in messages about the strongly held value of personal control. The media purports this value and denigrates those who struggle with it. Mothers may strongly believe in or may feel belittled by messages admonishing personal control. For example, messages about the link between personal control and obesity, particularly as delivered by healthcare providers, often target the adverse effects of obesity and the personal control needed to avoid this condition. As obesity is a common comorbidity among childbearing women in the USA, this message is delivered frequently to this population. For many women, this message is framed in personal failure rather than consideration of the SDoH that make nutritious eating out of economic reach and exercise difficult in dangerous neighborhoods. High crime neighborhoods with food deserts do not lend themselves to robust diet/exercise programs. On the other hand, appealing to personal control as a value can be empowering for those who have adequate resources, both financially and emotionally, to comply with recommendations of a healthy lifestyle.

Another example of operationalizing this value is making a birth plan. It demonstrates assumption of personal control in facing an unknown situation. It empowers the childbearing woman to express her desires and concerns for her baby and herself and to build partnership with her healthcare providers. A negative outcome can be a "failed" birth plan in which hopes and dreams are not realized, often out of the personal control of the mother. The sense of defeat can be bitter. There is also the situation where the birth plan attempts to subsume good clinical judgment and patient-provider partnership, sometimes at significant or life-threatening risk to either or both mother and baby. Personal control, as an American value, can have either positive or negative effects on maternal wellbeing and health outcomes.

1.3.3 Individualism

The value of individualism, idealized by the Founding Fathers, especially Benjamin Franklin (Franklin, 2013 orig 1732), it is in sharp relief to collectivist values in other cultures (Nisbett, 2004). It implies the primacy and autonomy of the individual and the need for personal freedom, especially as it relates to liberty of conscience. Deeply embedded in American folk psychology, individualism permeates the social milieu from the nuclear family structure and childrearing approaches to tensions about individual rights versus larger community rights. This premier American value has been noted by almost every writer on the American character, including Bellah et al. (1996) and Robert Putnam (2000). This value has been shown to weaken in times of individual, family, or community stress (Bianchi, 2016) and even historical promoters of American individualism are credited with expressing some reticence to absolute individualism. The widely quoted proverb, "Your liberty to swing your fist ends just where my nose begins" has been attributed, without strong evidence, to Founding Father John Adams, Oliver Wendell Holmes, John Stuart Mill, and Abraham Lincoln.

Individualism, as a cultural value in influencing decisions and maternal health outcomes, is exemplified in three of the most contentious contemporary issues within American society. The first is exposure of childbearing women to COVID-19 by the unvaccinated population. Another is COVID-19 vaccination uptake among childbearing women themselves. Third is the American woman's legal and constitutional right to pregnancy termination as defined by *Roe v. Wade* (Roe v. Wade, 1973). This right, currently either fully enacted or restricted, depending upon regional statutes, is approached from both perspectives by arguments centering on the value of individualism. These issues have the potential to profoundly affect maternal health outcomes.

1.3.4   Action-Orientation

Action-orientation, as opposed to state-orientation, is the inclination to act deliberatively in a situation in contrast to accepting the status quo or allowing events to happen without intervention. Action-orientation values proactive decisions in a situation, embracing a worldview that allows the use of personal power to make changes (Kuhl, 1981, 1985, 1994). This value is quickly operationalized in evaluating situations of danger (Koole & van den Berg, 2005). Conversely, state-orientation embraces a worldview that defines events as unfolding without much hope of change, even with effort, and may speak to unchangeable destiny as a driving force (Kuhl, 1994).

As a corollary of action-orientation, Americans typically idealize hard work, often defined as physical labor but more recently as mental or emotional work as well (Allemand, et al. 2008; Fernando et al., 2014; Harmon-Jones & Harmon-Jones, 2002). It includes deliberative action in both employment and personal spaces and is admonished with the expression: "Put your shoulder to the wheel." To other societies, Americans may appear intense in their commitment to long hours of employment, efforts to maximize financial gains, and choosing to spend personal leisure time in improvement of their personal space (De Vaus & McAllister, 1991; Halman & Müller, 2006; Jiang et al., 2014).

The cultural value of action-orientation can be both negative and positive for decisions affecting maternal health outcomes. Health education messages during pre- and postnatal care often stress deliberative action by the mother to protect her health and the health of her growing baby. These messages assume a worldview that personal actions can affect outcome. Most American mothers accept this message of cause and effect, but not all. The first author recalls a client, a pregnant woman who lived in poverty, without adequate transportation, nutrition, and income for a sustainable life. The woman did what she could to care for herself within her limited economic situation, but at 24 weeks gestation, her preterm baby was stillborn. The mother was heartbroken, but did not attribute the loss of a beloved and desired child to the SDoH afflicting her life. Her words to me (BA) were, "This baby was not of this world. It was not her fate to live." Another mother, who I attended in birth, delivered a preterm baby. She was a recent immigrant, having survived horrendous genocidal experiences. This mother spoke of karma, surrendering emotionally to the loss of the baby. She did give her a beautiful, culturally-appropriate name for the next incarnation, but did not want to nurse the baby. With guidance from the neonatal intensive care unit (NICU) nurses, she agreed to try to provide breast milk. I went with her to the NICU every day to encourage her with lactation. Her tough little girl was determined to live. Now she is a thriving young woman with a proud mother who decided that sometimes deliberative action can make a difference.

Tensions can be severe when expectant management and support for physiologic birth conflicts with action-oriented technological intervention in hope of protecting or speeding up the birth process. There are gradations from thoughtful, responsible care within the framework of respectful childbirth to abuse and violation of rights (Lalonde et al., 2019). These clinical decisions are frequently contextualized within the value system of the culture (United Nations, 2019).

1.3.5 Practicality

Practicality values efficient, realistic, and cost-effective ways of managing resources with productivity and the "bottom-line" maximized. "Time is money" and machines and people are expected to function well. Technology is revered. People are expected to work quickly, efficiently, set priorities, and be succinct in communication. Practicality exists in the here and now, critical of wasting time on activities with limited practical value. Idle daydreaming, contemplation, or even abstract thinking may be viewed as "wool-gathering" and not being in the "real world." Kahneman (2011) speaks to this dichotomy in his work *Thinking Fast and Slow*. Americans are generally regarded as a practical people, efficient, open to innovation, and willing to work hard to create rapid change (Hofstede, 1977; Metcalf et al., 2013; Yang & Gamble, 2013). Practicality leads to a "can-do" mentality exemplified by folk heroes like Rosie the Riveter, a World War II symbol of practicality. The media, popular culture, and the internet superhighway provide guidance and recommendations on how to be a practical person (see, https://learnlocal.org.au/10-practical-tips-on-being-more-effective-every-day/; edium.com/darius-foroux/four-books-that-will-turn-you-into-a-practical-thinker-bc62062b31c3).

In the USA, high technology often drives the childbearing process. The high cesarean section rate is an example of a quick solution when expectant management, trusting the birthing process, and adequate supportive care could have resulted in less intervention. Sometimes, it is easier and more efficient to use a surgical approach as opposed to gentle, time-consuming supportive care to encourage the birth to occur in its own time. Of course, there are emergency situations where practicality and quick decision-making are essential to the health of the mother and the baby. However, there is good evidence of routinized over-use of technology, not only cesarean section but also other interventions that restrict fluid, nutrition, and mobility during labor. These interventions are not always evidence-based, very expensive, and may be emotionally traumatic to the mother and her family.

1.3.6   Self-Reliance

Self-reliance views the individual as an autonomous, self-sufficient person expected to take responsibility for actions and succeed in life without undue dependence upon others. It is sometimes referred to as "bootstrapping" or DIY (do it yourself). It was idealized by Founding Father Benjamin Franklin who said, "God helps those who help themselves" (Franklin, 2013, orig 1732) and American philosopher Ralph Waldo Emerson in his work entitled, *Self-Reliance* (Kateb, 1995).

Self-reliance is a value that can build confidence in the ability to negotiate the challenges of life. It is frequently expected of oneself and others in the American society (Schaumberg & Flynn, 2017). An economically successful person may be lauded for adherence to this value (Galtung, 1986) even though many affluent people inherit their wealth. Lack of self-reliance is strongly condemned within the American culture (Lane, 2001).

The expectation of self-reliance can be overwhelming when one needs help. Sometimes, people excuse themselves or others for failing to be self-reliant when it is clearly impossible, as in sustaining a serious accident, but the cultural expectation is to strive for self-reliance even under very difficult circumstances (Galtung, 1981; Huberfield & Roberts, 2016; Quick et al., 1992). Former first lady Michelle Obama metaphorically spoke of extending a ladder to help people up when total bootstrapping is not possible.

A substance-abusing mother may be described as lacking in coping skills and self-reliance in the management of her life. She might actually tell a different story—that self-medicating is the way that she can be self-reliant, not depending upon others for her emotional wellbeing or her medication supply from persons with legal prescriptive authority. In either case, the value of self-reliance is being expressed.

Many first-time parents, lacking fine-tuned child-care skills, seek to learn about the formidable responsibilities of parenting so that they can feel confidently self-reliant. They also seek to be perceived by significant others, such as grandparents, their healthcare providers, and their community circle as mastering the art of parental self-reliance.

1.4   Summary

The overarching, dominant cultural values of the nation are widely disseminated and generally understood, even if not always adhered to or shared. They are reflected in the history, stories, and myths of a people. They have tremendous power to shape thinking, often used as the standard for explaining national character, lauding persons held in high regard, and ostracizing those less positively viewed.

This work examines five key American cultural values that have the potential to impact maternal health outcomes. Using an interdisciplinary critical analysis approach, it examines cultural expression, value-driven decision-making, and resource distribution within the context of the maternal health and the markers of national health defined in the SDoH.

References

Alemán, J., & Woods, D. (2016). Value orientations from the world values survey: How comparable are they cross-nationally? *Comparative Political Studies, 49*(8), 1039–1067. https://doi.org/10.1177/0010414015600458

Allemand, M., Job, V., Christen, S., & Keller, M. (2008). Forgivingness and action orientation. *Personality and Individual Differences, 45*(8), 762–766.

Amankwaa, L. C., Records, K., Kenner, C., Roux, G., Stone, S. E., & Walker, D. S. (2018). African-American mothers' persistent excessive maternal death rates. *Nursing Outlook, 66*(3), 316–318.

Bandura, A. (1982). Self-efficacy mechanism in human agency. *American Psychologist, 37*(2), 122–147.

Bandura, A. (1986). *Social foundations of thought and action: A social cognitive theory.* Prentice-Hall.

Bandura, A. (1989). Human agency in social cognitive theory. *American Psychologist, 44*(9), 1175–1184.

Bandura, A. (1997). *Self-efficacy: The exercise of control.* W.H. Freeman and Company.

Baumeister, R. F. (2015). Conquer yourself conquer the world. *Scientific American, 312*(4), 60–65.

Bellah, R., Sullivan, W., Tipton, S., Madsen, R., & Swidler, A. (1996). *Habits of the heart: Individualism and commitment in American life.* University of California Press.

Bianchi, E. C. (2016). American individualism rises and falls with the economy: Cross-temporal evidence that individualism declines when the economy falters. *Journal of Personality and Social Psychology, 111*(4), 567.

Brunson, J., & Suh, S. (2020). Behind the measures of maternal and reproductive health: Ethnographic accounts of inventory and intervention. *Social Science & Medicine, 254*, 112730.

Centers for Disease Control and Prevention. (2020). *Pregnancy mortality surveillance system: Trends in pregnancy-related deaths.* Centers for Disease Control and Prevention. Retrieved December 9, 2021 from https://www.cdc.gov/reproductivehealth/maternal-mortality/pregnancy-mortality-surveillance-system.htm#trends

Central Intelligence Agency. (2021). *The World Factbook: United States, People and Society.* Retrieved December 21 from https://www.cia.gov/the-world-factbook/countries/united-states/#people-and-society

Cusimano, C., & Goodwin, G. P. (2020). People judge others to have more voluntary control over beliefs than they themselves do. *Journal of Personality and Social Psychology, 119*(5), 999–1029.

Davis, N. L., Smoots, A. N., & Goodman, D. A. (2019). Pregnancy-related deaths: Data from 14 U.S. maternal mortality review committees, 2008-2017. https://www.cdc.gov/reproductivehealth/maternal-mortality/erase-mm/MMR-Data-Brief_2019-h.pdf

De Tocqueville, A. (2003). *Democracy in America. Translated by Gerald Bevan from French original 1835–1840.* Penguin Classics.

De Vaus, D., & McAllister, I. (1991). Gender and work orientation: Values and satisfaction in Western Europe. *Work and Occupations, 18*(1), 72–93. https://doi.org/10.1177/0730888491018001004

Fernando, J. W., Kashima, Y., & Laham, S. M. (2014). Multiple emotions: A person-centered approach to the relationship between intergroup emotion and action orientation. *Emotion, 14*(4), 722–732.

Franklin, B. (1949). In M. Farrand (Ed.), *The autobiography of Benjamin Franklin: A restoration of a "fair copy"*. University of California Press.

Franklin, B. (1961). *The autobiography and other writings*. Signet.

Franklin, B. (2013). In B. Blaisdell (Ed.), *(Original date 1732) poor Richard's Almanack and other writings*. Dover Publications, Inc.

Galla, B. M., & Duckworth, A. L. (2015). More than resisting temptation: Beneficial habits mediate the relationship between self-control and positive life outcomes. *Journal of Personality and Social Psychology, 109*(3), 508–525.

Galtung, J. (1981). The politics of self-reliance. In H. Muñoz (Ed.), *From dependency to development: Strategies to overcome underdevelopment and inequality* (p. 24). Taylor and Francis.

Galtung, J. (1986). In search of self-reliance. In P. Elkins (Ed.), *The living economy: A new economics in the making* (p. 13). Taylor and Francis.

Glasser, W. (1985). *Control theory: A new explanation of how we control our lives*. Harper and Row.

Goncalves, A. S., Ferreira, I. M., Pestana-Santos, M., Prata, A. P., & McCourt, C. (2020). Antenatal care policies for low-risk pregnant women in high-income countries with a universal health system: A scoping review protocol. *JBI Evidence Synthesis, 18*, 1537.

Halman, L., & Müller, H. (2006). Contemporary work values in Africa and Europe: Comparing orientations to work in African and European societies. *International Journal of Comparative Sociology, 47*(2), 117–143. https://doi.org/10.1177/0020715206065381

Harmon-Jones, E., & Harmon-Jones, C. (2002). Testing the action-based model of cognitive dissonance: The effect of action orientation on postdecisional attitudes. *Personality and Social Psychology Bulletin, 28*(6), 711–723. https://doi.org/10.1177/0146167202289001

Healthy People. (2030). U.S. Department of Health and Human Services, Office of Disease Prevention and Health Promotion. https://health.gov/healthypeople/objectives-and-data/social-determinants-health

Hofstede, G. (1977). *Culture's consequences: International differences in work-related values* (Vol. 5).

Hoyert, D. L. (2021). Maternal mortality rates in the United States, 2019 (Health E-stats 2021, Issue). https://www.cdc.gov/nchs/data/hestat/maternal-mortality-2021/E-Stat-Maternal-Mortality-Rates-H.pdf

Huberfeld, N., & Roberts, J. L. (2016). Health care and the myth of self-reliance. *BCL Rev., 57*, 1–60.

Infurna, F. J., Ram, N., & Gerstorf, D. (2013). Level and change in perceived control predict 19-year mortality: Findings from the Americans' changing lives study. *Developmental Psychology, 49*(10), 1833–1847. https://doi.org/10.1037/a0031041

Jiang, Y., Zhan, L., & Rucker, D. D. (2014). Power and action orientation: Power as a catalyst for consumer switching behavior. *Journal of Consumer Research, 41*(1), 183–196.

Kahneman, D. (2011). *Thinking, fast and slow*. Macmillan.

Kateb, G. (1995). *Emerson and Self-reliance*. Sage.

Kelley, A. (2020). *Public health evaluation and the social determinants of health*. Routledge.

Kenner, C., Ashford, K., Badr, L. K., Black, B., Bloch, J., Mainous, R., McGrath, J., Premji, S., Sinclair, S., & Terhaar, M. (2018). American Academy of Nursing on policy: Reducing preterm births in the United States: Maternal infant health, child, adolescent and family, and women's health expert panels (August 13, 2018). *Nursing Outlook, 66*, 499.

Koblinsky, M., Chowdhury, M. E., Moran, A., & Ronsmans, C. (2012). Maternal morbidity and disability and their consequences: Neglected agenda in maternal health. *Journal of Health, Population, and Nutrition, 30*(2), 124.

Koblinsky, M., Moyer, C. A., Calvert, C., Campbell, J., Campbell, O. M., Feigl, A. B., Graham, W. J., Hatt, L., Hodgins, S., & Matthews, Z. (2016). Quality maternity care for every woman, everywhere: A call to action. *The Lancet, 388*(10057), 2307–2320. https://www.thelancet.com/journals/lancet/article/PIIS0140-6736(16)31333-2/fulltext

Koole, S. L., & Van den Berg, A. E. (2005). Lost in the wilderness: Terror management, action orientation, and nature evaluation. *Journal of Personality and Social Psychology, 88*(6), 1014–1028.

Kuhl, J. (1981). Motivational and functional helplessness: The moderating effect of state versus action orientation. *Journal of Personality and Social Psychology, 40*(1), 155–170.

Kuhl, J. (1985). Volitional mediators of cognition-behavior consistency: Self-regulatory processes and action versus state orientation. In *Action control* (pp. 101–128). Springer.

Kuhl, J. (1994). A theory of self-regulation: Action versus state orientation, self-discrimination, and some applications. *Applied Psychology, 41*(2), 97–129.

Lalonde, A., Herschderfer, K., Pascali-Bonaro, D., Hanson, C., Fuchtner, C., & Visser, G. H. (2019). The international childbirth initiative: 12 steps to safe and respectful MotherBaby–family maternity care. *International Journal of Gynecology & Obstetrics, 146*(1), 65–73.

Lane, R. E. (2001). Self-reliance and empathy: The enemies of poverty—And of the poor. *Political Psychology, 22*(3), 473–492.

Larroca, S. G.-T., Valera, F. A., Herrera, E. A., Hernandez, I. C., Lopez, Y. C., & De Leon-Luis, J. (2020). Human development index of the maternal country of origin and its relationship with maternal near miss: A systematic review of the literature. *BMC Pregnancy and Childbirth, 20*(1), 1–24.

Lerner, M. J. (1980). *The belief in a just world: A fundamental delusion*. Plenum.

MacDorman, M. F., & Declercq, E. (2018). The failure of United States maternal mortality reporting and its impact on women's lives [article]. *Birth: Issues in Perinatal Care, 45*(2), 105–108. https://doi.org/10.1111/birt.12333

Mehta, L. S., Sharma, G., Creanga, A. A., Hameed, A. B., Hollier, L. M., Johnson, J. C., Leffert, L., McCullough, L. D., Mujahid, M. S., & Watson, K. (2021). Call to action: Maternal health and saving mothers: A policy statement from the American Heart Association. *Circulation, 144*(15), e251–e269.

Metcalf, S., Kamarainen, A., Grotzer, T., & Dede, C. (2013). Teacher perceptions of the practicality and effectiveness of immersive ecological simulations as classroom curricula. *International Journal of Virtual and Personal Learning Environments (IJVPLE), 4*(3), 66–77.

Mirowsky, J., & Ross, C. E. (2007). Life course trajectories of perceived control and their relationship to education. *American Journal of Sociology, 112*(5), 1339–1382.

National Center for Health Statistics. (2021). Healthy People 2020 Progress Table. *Healthy People 2020 Final Review*. https://doi.org/10.15620/cdc:111173

National Research Council and the Institute of Medicine. (2013). *U.S. health in international perspective: Shorter lives, poorer health*. The National Academies Press.

Nisbett, R. (2004). *The geography of thought: How Asians and westerners think differently... And why*. Simon and Schuster.

Petersen, E., Lightner, S., & Baksh, L. (2021). *Pregnancy related deaths*. Centers for Disease Control and Prevention. Retrieved 12-9-21 from https://www.cdc.gov/reproductivehealth/maternal-mortality/preventing-pregnancy-related-deaths.html

Putnam, R. (2000). *Bowling alone: The collapse and revival of American community*. Simon & Schuster.

Quick, J. C., Joplin, J. R., Nelson, D. L., & Quick, J. D. (1992). Behavioral responses to anxiety: Self-reliance, counterdependence, and overdependence. *Anxiety, Stress, and Coping, 5*(1), 41–54.

Roe v.Wade, 410 U.S. 113 (1973).

Rotter, J. B. (1966). Generalized expectancies for internal versus external control of reinforcement. *Psychological Monographs: General and Applied, 80*(1), 1.

Ryon, H. S., & Gleason, M. E. (2018). Reciprocal support and daily perceived control: Developing a better understanding of daily support transactions across a major life transition. *Journal of Personality and Social Psychology, 115*(6), 1034.

Schaumberg, R., & Flynn, F. (2017). Self-reliance: A gender perspective on its relationship to communality and leadership evaluations. *Academy of Management Journal, 60*(5), 1859–1881. https://doi.org/10.5465/amj.2015.0018

Thompson-Dudiak, M. (2021). The Black maternal health crisis: How to right a harrowing history through judicial and legislative reform. *DePaul Journal for Social Justice, 14*, 1.

Tikkanen, R., Gunja, M. Z., FitzGerald, M., & Zephyrin, L. (2020). *Maternal mortality and maternity care in the United States compared to 10 other developed countries*. Issue briefs.

United Health Foundation. (2021). America's health rankings: Health of women and children. *United Health Foundation.*. https://www.americashealthrankings.org/explore/health-of-women-and-children/measure/maternal_mortality/state/ALL

United Nations. (2019). *A human rights-based approach to mistreatment and violence against women in reproductive health services with a focus on childbirth and obstetric violence* (advancement of women, Issue. U. Nations. https://digitallibrary.un.org/record/3823698

United Nations Human Rights Council. (2018). *Report of the Special Rapporteur on extreme poverty and human rights on his mission to the United States of America*. Retrieved from https://digitallibrary.un.org/record/1629536/files/A_HRC_38_33_Add-EN.pdf

Villines, Z. (2019). The maternal mortality lie that ensures women will keep dying. *Daily KOS*. https://www.dailykos.com/stories/2019/10/23/1894584/-The-Maternal-Mortality-Lie-That-Ensures-Women-Will-Keep-Dying

Weil, A., & Reichert, A. (2021). *Reversing the US maternal mortality crisis: A report of the Aspen health strategy group* (the Aspen Institute, Issue. T. A. Institute. https://www.aspeninstitute.org/publications/reversing-the-u-s-maternal-mortality-crisis/

World Health Organization. (2019). Trends in maternal mortality 2000 to 2017: Estimates by WHO, UNICEF, UNFPA, World Bank Group and the United Nations Population Division (ISBN 978–92–4-151648-8). WHO. https://www.who.int/data/gho/data/themes/topics/sdg-target-3-1-maternal-mortality

Yang, Y., & Gamble, J. (2013). Effective and practical critical thinking-enhanced EFL instruction. *ELT Journal, 67*(4), 398–412.

Chapter 2
Cultural Values as a Basis for Decision-Making

Eugene N. Anderson and Barbara A. Anderson

2.1 Maternal Health Outcomes: A Reflection of Decisions

Maternal health outcomes reflect decisions about maternal health and wellbeing made at all levels within a nation. These decisions may result in positive and negative outcomes. They are grounded in the moral foundations, history, traditions, and cultural values of a nation. American cultural values are a strong driver in decisions that operates from the individual, family, and community levels to national policy.

Maternal health in the United States (USA) does not compare favorably to other high income countries (Weil & Reichert, 2021; World Health Organization [WHO], 2019). While not exclusively so, poor outcomes disproportionally reflect health disparities and less privileged mothers in the nation (Hoyert, 2021). The question is *why* do these poor outcomes persist in a very affluent country. Examining the process by which decisions affecting maternal health are made is a beginning step in answering this question. This chapter explores the theoretical foundations of decision-making and cultural values that can drive decision-making.

2.2 Theoretical Foundations of Decision-Making

Decision-making is the study of the allocation of limited resources among conflicting purposes. Some decisions are relatively straightforward (e.g., the individual decision to brush one's teeth versus facing tooth decay, providing one has access to

E. N. Anderson (✉)
University of California, Riverside, CA, USA

B. A. Anderson
Frontier Nursing University, Versailles, KY, USA

© The Author(s), under exclusive license to Springer Nature Switzerland AG 2023 17
B. A. Anderson, L. R. Roberts (eds.), *Maternal Health and American Cultural Values*, Global Maternal and Child Health, https://doi.org/10.1007/978-3-031-23969-4_2

a toothbrush or other tool, such as eucalyptus twigs). Other decisions are agonizing, requiring enormous discussion about resource allocation. An example is governmental budgeting decisions. Every act from individual to collective level involves due consideration, even if purely subconscious. Subconscious attention in decision-making is particularly valuable as it allows us to attend to cues in our environment even when not focusing on them (de Becker, 1998; Gigerenzer, 2007; Gladwell, 2005). Routinized decisions, such as getting up or eating breakfast at a specific time, makes life easier and demands minimal attention. Many decisions, however, require significant attention and time.

2.2.1   The Study of Decision-Making

Studies of decision-making are an important research domain in economics, anthropology and the social sciences (Gladwin, 1989). The basis of this work is the perception that individuals usually act on the basis of considered decisions, based upon knowledge. In order to make a decision, one must be cognizant of the options, the likely outcomes of a choice, and what factors to consider. If knowledge is certain, decisions are usually easy, but knowledge is often imperfect and uncertain. Sometimes there is no way to know and decisions are made based upon the best available knowledge and hope.

Researchers ask detailed questioning in capturing the sequential steps in making a decision. They query informants about the process as it leads to a particular decision. Examples are when and what crops to plant (Gladwin, 1989), what to do when someone in the family is sick (Young & Garro, 1994; Anderson [published under Frye], 1995), or how to fish sustainably (Aswani & Weiant, 2004).

Christina Gladwin's classic work (1989) involved agricultural crop choice. Another classic study, with methodological reflections, is *Medical Choice in a Mexican Village* (Young & Garro, 1994). Frye (1995) described algorithms used by Cambodian refugee women, who were culturally acknowledged in the family health guardian role. These algorithms describe how the women decided who received healthcare and under what conditions it was traditional or allopathic care. Aswani and Weiant (2004) went beyond economic and biological methods in fishing research to a thoughtful analysis of how decisions are made for sustainability. This line of questioning is foundational, explaining *who, what, when, where*, and *how much* is involved in a decision.

This questioning technique assumes that decisions can be broken down into ordered sequences of yes/no answers: Can I get the seed for this crop? Can I get fertilizer for it? Can I get enough water for it? It assumes that making a complex decision involves a series of yes/no decisions to form a *decision tree* or an *algorithm*. In clear-cut matters, one can usually break down decisions into yes vs. no or more vs. less choices. Sometimes when it appears that an individual is acting on impulse, when, in fact, he is subconsciously integrating several pieces of knowledge simultaneously. Careful sequential questioning allows the researcher to facilitate the process, expand information through in-depth interviewing, and formulate a decision tree analysis.

It is a powerful technique for decisions that involve known, important and routine choices with a good knowledge base, important consequences, and fairly clear-cut answers. Examples are the management of cardio-pulmonary arrest or whether to introduce a new agricultural crop. For instance, an experienced gardener normally knows exactly what crops she can plant in her environment, the conditions of the soil, and whom to ask for further information. Another example affecting everyday life is the decision about what toothpaste to use. One observes the price, asks others in his social circle and/or his dentist for recommendations, and may even taste the toothpaste. Other factors in the final decision might include the appearance of the tube and marketing claims. However, in new, unforeseen, and emergency situations, knowledge base may be less definitive, consequences unknown or unforeseen, and credible information sources unclear. Public response to the COVID-19 pandemic demonstrates a complex situation in which many persons find decision-making very difficult.

In short, decision-making research is designed to find out how decisions are made. In practice, this means asking informants what they do in given situations. Then one asks why they do so. This often produces unhelpful results: "I've never thought about it," "we always do it that way," "everybody does that." Such answers require further observation and questioning, to watch what people actually do. They almost always have alternatives: *We usually do it this way, but we can do it this other way.* The researchers then asks: Why did you pick Choice A instead of B? Informants may or may not be clear about why they do it a certain way.

Some decisions are simple: "I got that toothpaste because it was the cheapest in the store." However, if a rural hospital has a high caesarian section rate, difficult and involved decisions may not be apparent until it becomes evident the only obstetrician in the county is in the hospital one day a week, the nursing workforce is highly understaffed, and there are no nurse-midwives in the country available to support physiological birth (Hung et al., 2016; Seigel, 2018). Young and Garro (1994) found that in poverty-stricken Michoacan, Mexican villagers preferred allopathic care at a clinic or hospital, but rarely had the money. They would borrow money and go without food or other necessities for a few days. They also knew a range of traditional practices, garden and wild-gathered herbs with medicinal value, magical practices, and prayer, as well as basic first aid. They balanced these traditional remedies according to knowledge about effectiveness of care compared to allopathic care. This decision-making process involved a complex mixture of economic calculation, values, and personal preferences.

2.2.2 Cultural Alternatives in Decision-Making

Studies of decision-making have proven conclusively that people do not just mindlessly follow the rules of their culture. Cultures require survival and adaptation. Every culture provides alternative solutions for almost any situation. Even strictly within their cultural rules, people are forced to consider multiple choices all the time. These decisions usually involve a certain amount of risk and uncertainty. "I shot an arrow into the air. It fell to earth I knew not where." (Longfellow, 2015).

To reduce uncertainty, people search for information. The cost of getting this information is often the greatest cost and source of distress in making decisions. It involves constructing different models. An example is a single-factor economic model is one in which the person making the decision opts for the cheapest option. "Cheapness" may not be strictly monetary; it may involve the least time-consuming option, the least physical effort, the most accessible option, or the solution that requires no further effort.

Most models are more complex. There are trade-offs in emotional satisfaction, fun, social obligations, desires for control, and compliance with cultural messages as well as economic solutions. All factors being equal, people tend to decide based upon prior knowledge and cultural sensitivities, sometimes missing the chance to learn quicker, easier, or more efficient ways. Sometimes, they decide impulsively deciding that the cost of acquiring full information is simply too much effort. Usually, however, people weigh their choices, including all those alternatives provided within their culture and sometimes stretch the culture to expand alternatives. Culture is not a strait-jacket. It helps to define a set of possible, practical, and often creative choices. In his biography *Steve Jobs*, Walter Isaacson (2011) describes the famed Apple cofounder as having the skill to expand cultural alternatives.

The result of such modeling is cost-benefit analysis: how people calculate the benefits versus the costs of getting them. These costs are not solely financial. They may be emotional or social. Even the apparently "cheapest" models can be complicated, the financial cost and benefits balanced against cost and benefit to one's emotional, spiritual, and social self. The values of the culture speak to these issues and such decisions are not made in isolation of the culture. People make decisions with those they trust within their culture and those who guide them in the path of cultural knowledge. One of the most profound examples cultural guiding is the story of the two wolves.

Box 2.1 The Story of the Two Wolves
"My child, it's time to teach you the most important lesson about life and people. It is that everyone has within two wolves: a good wolf that wants to help everyone and do what's best for all, and a bad wolf that wants to do evil and hurt people and the world." "Father, that's scary. It really worries me. Which wolf wins out in the end?" asked the child. The father replied," "The wolf you feed." *Native American folktale* (Anderson & Anderson, 2021. p. ix)

2.3 Cultural Models: Guide to Decision-Making

Decision-making studies have led to scholars in developing cultural models of how to act appropriately or what to expect (cf. Frake in Dil, 1980). There are cultural models of greeting ("Hello, how are you?") or expressing sympathy ("I'm so sorry to hear that."). Cooking recipes are cultural models as are plans and expectations for celebrating holidays. Serious scholarship on cultural modeling has emerged, including specific instructions on how to conduct this research and analyze the findings (Kronenfeld, 2008). There are excellent examples of research utilizing cultural modeling including notable contributions by Victor de Munck (2011), Giovanni Bernnardo, Naomi Quinn, Claudia Strauss, Bradd Shore, and others (Kronenfeld et al., 2011).

2.3.1 Norms and Values

Cultural models orient people morally and emotionally as well as cognitively. They are expressed in *norms* and *values*. Norms are rules for behavior with the expectation that behavior will follow a prescribed cultural model. Norms can range from simple and automatic, like greeting rituals, to highly complex. They can change fairly rapidly. For example, the standard American greeting ritual "Hello, how are you?" has added "Have a nice day!" within the last few decades. Norms remain somewhat understudied, despite their obvious importance.

Far better studied are values, broad principles for orienting one's life. These are much less apt to be simple. They involve valuing the natural environment or seeing it as something to be "tamed" and destroyed; valuing human life or regarding it as expendable; valuing hallowed traditions or seeing them as an intolerable restraint. Values are generally thought to be moral, and moral rules are values, but this is relative. Such things as valuing promptness and efficient use of time are less morally compelling than valuing human life. Morals and values are, in turn, based on ethical principles.

Anthropologists have been seriously studying values since the 1950s. An epochal book for launching this research was *Variations in Value Orientations* by Florence Kluckhohn and Floyd Strodtbeck (1961). They, with Clyde Kluckhohn, John Whiting, Kimball Romney, and others, studied values of different ethnic groups in New Mexico (Vogt, 1966). These studies encompass values relating to time, space, and person. These values were expressed historically in different ways by Hispanics, Mormon and Protestant settlers, and Native Americans. Particularly insightful anthropological studies examined Hopi (Brandt, 1954) and Navaho values and ethics (cf. Brandt, and Ladd 1957).

2.3.2 Decisions and Cultural Values

Decisions are inevitably grounded in cultural values. These are embedded in moral foundations, beliefs, and traditions. Values complicate decision-making, especially when two values run counter to each other. Values often involve choice between narrow, short-term interests and wide, long-term ones. The normal human tendency is to overvalue the former, on the proverbial theory that a bird in the hand is worth two in the bush (Gigerenzer 2007; Kahneman 2011). Saving on healthcare in the short term very often leads to enormously greater costs in the long run. This is an example of *heuristics*: natural biases that may cause one to infer incorrect conclusions without adequate consideration. Another common heuristic is exposure to information. If one has been reading many articles recently or hearing about a particular group committing crimes, it will lead to suspicion of persons from that population group. This bias may occur even as one understands that this information is not consistent with the wide, long-term profile of this group. The conflict between noble principles of sharing and short-term material acquisition can be phrased as competition between need and greed. However, the salient point is that decisions are about allocating resources among competing ends. The result is that values are not fixed rules. They are interpreted within specific context that may require negotiation (Bourdieu 1977).

When decisions are being made and there is difference in interpretation, negotiating the meaning of the specific cultural values can lead to conflict. This conflict can be driven by assumptions of how "worthy" or "deserving" specific persons or groups are. At worst, people may be dehumanized, such as occurs in genocide (Anderson & Anderson, 2021; Smith 2011, 2020, 2021). Nobel Prize winner, economist, and philosopher Amartya Sen sums up much of this conflict in his theory of social choice (Sen, 2018). Social choice involves rectifying divergent interests and concerns. This process requires widespread public communication and reasonable standards with majority rule among populations that share cultural values and norms (Sen, 2018).

Reality, however, may be very different. Majority rule may not be present; it does not always work; and minorities are easily repressed. Resilience by minorities in the face of such repression does not imply they are free of suffering or abuse or have full social choice. Among mainstream populations without significant repression, there are also conditions of suffering and abuse that limit social choice. Cultural values frame how a society calculates social choice that includes personal well-being (the *affordances* of adequate food, shelter, safety, and healthcare) and personal freedom.

2.4 American Cultural Values

The US Constitution, drafted in 1787, describes core American cultural values. Subsequently, these values have been continually debated. Contemporary consideration of American cultural values is well described in the work of Jonathan Haidt

(2012) and the writing of Graham et al. *Mapping the Moral Domain* (2011). American cultural values influence decisions that influence social and environmental conditions affecting the health of the nation.

These decisions, made by individuals, communities, professional groups, and government, are mirrored in the health of mothers. This work is a critical analysis of five American cultural values that influence decisions around maternal health at all levels:

- Personal control.
- Individualism.
- Action-orientation.
- Practicality.
- Self-reliance.

2.4.1 Personal Control

From the perspective of decision-making, the cultural value of personal control embodies Sen's theory of social choice (2018). As described by Sen, there must be majority rule, standards deemed reasonable, and shared values for social choice to function in society. In addition, there must be public communication to rectify different ideologies of personal well-being and personal freedom (2018). A key example of cultural clash in the USA around the value of personal control is the public response to the COVID-19 pandemic. Controversy has surrounded public health decisions and recommendations. There has been mixed public response to personal control measures (masks and vaccines) to prevent exposure to and spread of the virus.

2.4.2 Individualism

Individualism implies autonomy. American individualism speaks to autonomy in terms of the uniqueness of each person, the right to opinions, liberty of conscience, and freedom of expression (Kohls, 1984). It is a cherished value protected by the United States Bill of Rights, ratified in 1791 as an addition to the Constitution (https://www.archives.gov/founding-docs/bill-of-rights/what-does-it-say). Perhaps more than any of the values selected for this work, it supports the personal freedom of each American.

Individualism implies the importance of the individual in contrast to collectivist values. As such, the expression of this value may lead to conflict about rights: where do my rights stop and yours start? Decisions about fetal rights and maternal rights, if they are in conflict, center on this value. Federal law, per Supreme Court decision in Roe vs. Wade, formerly protected maternal autonomy and individual decision-making about pregnancy continuation, but has now been overturned. Regional statutes, third-party payers, and institutional policies have placed restrictions around individual decision-making, not only for the pregnant person but also for healthcare providers. Different ideologies of personal well-being and personal freedom (see Sen, 2018) drive the debate and the implementation of federal law at local and state levels.

2.4.3 Action-Orientation

The cultural value of action-orientation encourages pro-active decision-making to make change. It encourages the use of personal power in making change (Kuhl, 1994). When there are differing views of what action needs to happen and who makes the decision, social choice theory speaks to rectifying divergent interests and concerns with acknowledgement of shared values, appropriate use of power, and attention to well-being (Sen, 2018).

Action-oriented decision-making about maternal health can lead to swiftly-implemented changes that diminish risk and save the lives of mothers. An example is the development of systematic protocols (*safety bundles*) for managing obstetrical emergencies (The Council on Patient Safety in Women's Health Care, 2018). (See https://safehealthcareforeverywoman.org/patient-safety-bundles/).

Conversely, the value of action-orientation can lead to distress when a person values personal control and individualism but feels powerless to influence action in decision-making. The risk is greatest for those who have less personal freedom and well-being (Fernando, Kashima, & Laham, 2014; Harmon-Jones & Harmon-Jones, 2002).

2.4.4 Practicality

Americans highly value and are expected to be practical. History speaks to many practical inventions encouraged by this cultural ethos. The innovation and hard work of Americans is legendary (Metcalf et al., 2013; Yang & Gamble, 2013). While highly productive economically, this value may interfere the time needed for deep analysis and creative thinking (Kahneman, 2011) or for attending to human needs.

Economics and practicality can drive thinking about attention needed in caring for the sick, weak, and frail. It can undercut proposals to support family development, such as family leave, child care credits, community-based mental health programs, and postpartum home visiting. In some cases, practicality ends up costing more in the long run and can contribute to poorer maternal outcomes (Kozhimannil, et al. 2015). An example is the widespread closure of maternity care services, especially in rural areas, related to inadequate staffing (Hung et al., 2016; Seigel 2018). More than 50% of rural hospitals in the USA no longer offer full-scope maternity services (Seigel, 2018). Conversely, decisions to implement community-based birth centers is in line with the cultural value of practicality that have improved maternal health outcomes. (Alliman, J., & Phillippi, J. 2016; Stapleton, S., Osborne, C., & Illuzzi, J., 2013).

2.4.5   Self-Reliance

Self-reliance views the individual as a self-managing human, able to take care of oneself without undue dependence upon on others. It is a strongly held value aimed at developing trust in one's ability to deal with the trials of everyday life. The ability to be self-reliant is encouraged in raising children. Not only is one expected to be self-reliant (Schaumberg & Flynn, 2017), but the failure to do so is highly criticized, even when facing seemingly impossible barriers like intransigent poverty (Lane, 2001).

The value of self-reliance can plays a powerful role in motivating one to make decisions to improve personal well-being. However, it can be daunting when facing difficulties, especially if isolated from community support (Huberfield & Roberts, 2016). Social and environmental conditions, the *social determinants of health*, can support or undermine health. These determinants are economic stability, education and healthcare access, quality of life in the community, and social cohesion (Healthy People, 2030). To be a healthy people, these social determinants all require cooperative community support (Healthy People, 2030).

Decisions influencing maternal healthcare are made with many considerations such as funding availability, provision of services, adequate staff to provide care, and acceptability. Minimal staffing in obstetrical units can lead to greater reliance upon technology-driven interventions and less direct human contact. The values of self-reliance and personal control can converge to create tensions in this low-touch situation. As described in the section on practicality, maternal health may be jeopardized by the decision to close formerly self-reliant hospitals. Maternity care deserts, such as those that exist in many rural areas in the USA, have very limited access to services and skilled maternal healthcare providers. At all levels, decisions to limit services and access contribute to poor maternal outcomes (Surgo Ventures, 2021).

2.5   Summary

Decisions about maternal health are made in the context of cultural values. This chapter describes a theoretical framework for decision-making and provides exemplars of value-driven decisions affecting maternal health outcomes within the American context. It explores five leading American cultural values with historic and ongoing influence that drive decision-making about maternal health.

References

Alliman, J., & Phillippi, J. (2016). Maternal outcomes in birth centers: An integrative review of the literature. *Journal of Midwifery and Women's Health, 61*(1), 21–51. https://doi.org/10.1111/jmwh.12356

Anderson, B. (Published under Frye, B). (1995). Use of cultural themes in promoting health among southeast Asian refugees. *American Journal of Health Promotion, 9*(4), 269–280.

Anderson, E., & Anderson, B. (2021). *Complying with genocide: The wolf you feed.* Lexington Books.

Aswani, S., & Weiant, P. (2004). Scientific evaluation in women's participatory management: Monitoring marine invertebrate refugia in the Solomon Islands. *Human Organization, 63,* 301–319.

Bourdieu, P. (1977). *Outline of a theory of practice.* Cambridge University Press.

Brandt, R. (1954). *Hopi ethics: A theoretical analysis.* University of Chicago Press.

De Becker, G. (1998). *The gift of fear: And other survival signals that protect us from violence.* Dell.

De Munck, V. (2011). Cognitive approaches to the study of romantic love: Semantic, cross-cultural, and as a process. In D. Kronenfeld, G. Bennardo, V. de Munck, & M. Fischer (Eds.), *A companion to cognitive anthropology* (p. 18). Wiley-Blackwell.

Dil, C. (1980). *Language and cultural description: Essays by Charles O. Frake.* Stanford University Press.

Fernando, J. W., Kashima, Y., & Laham, S. M. (2014). Multiple emotions: A person-centered approach to the relationship between intergroup emotion and action orientation. *Emotion, 14*(4), 722–732.

Gigerenzer, G. (2007). *Gut feelings: The intelligence of the unconscious.* Viking.

Gladwell, M. (2005). *Blink: The power of thinking without thinking.* Little.

Gladwin, C. (1989). *Ethnographic decision tree modeling.* Sage.

Graham, J., Nosek, B., Haidt, J., Iyer, R., Koleva, S., & Ditto, P. (2011). Mapping the moral domain. *Journal of Personality and Social Psychology, 101,* 366–385.

Haidt, J. (2012). *The righteous mind: Why good people are divided by politics and religion.* Pantheon Books.

Harmon-Jones, E., & Harmon-Jones, C. (2002). Testing the action-based model of cognitive dissonance: The effect of action orientation on postdecisional attitudes. *Personality and Social Psychology Bulletin, 28*(6), 711–723. https://doi.org/10.1177/0146167202289001

Health. (2030). U.S. Department of Health and Human Services, Office of Disease Prevention and Health Promotion. https://health.gov/healthypeople/objectives-and-data/social-determinants-health

Hoyert, D. (2021). *Maternal mortality rates in the United States, 2019* (health E-stats 2021, Issue. https://www.cdc.gov/nchs/data/hestat/maternal-mortality-2021/E-Stat-Maternal-Mortality-Rates-H.pdf

Huberfeld, N., & Roberts, J. L. (2016). Health care and the myth of self-reliance. *BCL Review, 57,* 1–60.

Hung, P., Kozhimannil, K., Casey, M., & Moscovice, I. (2016). Why are obstetric units in rural hospitals closing their doors? *Health Services Research, 51*(4), 1546–1560. https://doi.org/10.1111/1475-6773.12441

Isaacson, W. (2011). *Steve jobs: The exclusive biography.* Simon & Schuster.

Kahneman, D. (2011). *Thinking, fast and slow.* Farrar.

Kluckhohn, F., & Strodtbeck, F. (1961). *Variations in value orientations.* Row & Peterson.

Kohls, L. (1984). *The values Americans live by* (the Washington international center). https://www.fordham.edu/download/downloads/id/3193/values_americans_live_by.pdf

Kozhimannil, K., Casey, M., Hung, P., Han, X., Prasad, S., & Moscovice, I. (2015). The rural obstetric workforce in US hospitals: Challenges and opportunities. *Journal of Rural Health, 31*(4), 365–372. https://doi.org/10.1111/jrh.12112

Kronenfeld, D. (2008). *Culture, society, and cognition: Collective goals, values, action, and knowledge*. Mouiton de Gruyter.

Kronenfeld, D., Bennardo, G., de Munck, V., & Fischer, M. (2011). *A companion to cognitive anthropology*. Wiley-Blackwell.

Kuhl, J. (1994). A theory of self-regulation: Action versus state orientation, self-discrimination, and some applications. *Applied Psychology, 41*(2), 97–129.

Ladd, J. (1957). *The structure of a moral code: A philosophical analysis of ethical discourse applied to the ethics of the Indians*. Harvard University Press.

Lane, R. (2001). Self-reliance and empathy: The enemies of poverty—And of the poor. *Political Psychology, 22*(3), 473–492.

Longfellow, H. (2015). *The complete works of Henry Wadsworth Longfellow: The belfry of Bruges and other poems*. Palata Press.

Metcalf, S., Kamarainen, A., Grotzer, T., & Dede, C. (2013). Teacher perceptions of the practicality and effectiveness of immersive ecological simulations as classroom curricula. *International Journal of Virtual and Personal Learning Environments (IJVPLE), 4*(3), 66–77.

Schaumberg, R., & Flynn, F. (2017). Self-reliance: A gender perspective on its relationship to communality and leadership evaluations. *Academy of Management Journal, 60*(5), 1859–1881. https://doi.org/10.5465/amj.2015.0018

Sen, A. (2018). *Social choice and collective welfare: An expanded version*. Harvard University Press.

Seigel, J. (2018). *Delivering rural babies: Maternity care shortages in rural America*. (rural health voices. https://www.ruralhealthweb.org/blogs/ruralhealthvoices/march-2018/delivering-rural-babies-maternity-care-shortages

Smith, D. (2021). *Making monsters*. Harvard University Press.

Smith, D. (2020). *On inhumanity: Dehumanization and how to resist it*. Oxford University Press.

Smith, D. (2011). *Less than human: Why we demean, enslave and exterminate others*. St. Martin's Press.

Stapleton, S., Osborne, C., & Illuzzi, J. (2013). Outcomes of care in birth centers: Demonstration of a durable model. *Journal of Midwifery and Women's Health, 58*(1), 3–14. https://doi.org/10.1111/jmwh.12003

Surgo Ventures. (2021). *Getting hyperlocal to improve outcomes and achieve racial equity in maternal health: The US Maternal Vulnerability Index*. https://mvi.surgoventures.org/

The Council on Patient Safety in Women's Health Care. (2018). *Maternal Safety Bundles and Patient Safety Tools*. Retrieved from https://safehealthcareforeverywoman.org/patient-safety-bundles/

Vogt, E. (1966). *People of Rimrock: A study of five cultures*. Harvard University Press.

Weil, A., & Reichert, A. (2021). *Reversing the US maternal mortality crisis: A report of the Aspen health strategy group (the Aspen Institute, issue)*. T. A. Institute. https://www.aspeninstitute.org/publications/reversing-the-u-s-maternal-mortality-crisis/

World Health Organization. (2019). Trends in maternal mortality 2000 to 2017: Estimates by WHO, UNICEF, UNFPA, World Bank Group and the United Nations population division (ISBN 978–92–4-151648-8). WHO. https://www.who.int/data/gho/data/themes/topics/sdg-target-3-1-maternal-mortality

Yang, Y., & Gamble, J. (2013). Effective and practical critical thinking-enhanced EFL instruction. *ELT Journal, 67*(4), 398–412.

Young, J., & Garro, L. (1994). *Medical choice in a Mexican village* (2nd ed.). Westview.

Part II
The Lived Experience of American Mothers

Chapter 3
Social Regard for Motherhood

Lisa R. Roberts

3.1 Motherhood in the USA

Historically, the role of motherhood was defined by childbearing. However, advances of science in the 1800s brought about a shift in the American understanding of the role of mothers focusing more on child*rearing*, compared to child*bearing* (Doyle, 2018). In the early 1900s, being a mother was still considered women's major contribution to society. However, women's right to choose whether or not they wanted to be mothers began to gain public interest, despite lack of reproductive control available for most. Maternal mortality rates were extremely high. Scientific developments in medicine increased the possibility of timing pregnancies and limiting the number of children born, particularly for women with an economic advantage.

At the same time, the modern age of science created contradictory messaging for mothers. Mothers were to trust their instincts, yet told in minute detail how to take care of their children. They were admonished to consult a physician or other professional experts for education and scientific training on childrearing rather than relying on the counsel of older relatives. The mother-child dyad was still lauded as the best choice for a child's health and development. It was commonly understood that good mothers produced good children, while bad mothers produced bad children. Yet while mothers were to fully devote themselves to childrearing, changes in the American economy during and post-World War II (WWII) demanded that women join the formal workforce (paid work outside of the home), contributing to the race and class bias toward motherhood. Not only did women of color have less access to contraception, a distinction grew between working women and working mothers

L. R. Roberts (✉)
Loma Linda University, Loma Linda, CA, USA

© The Author(s), under exclusive license to Springer Nature Switzerland AG 2023
B. A. Anderson, L. R. Roberts (eds.), *Maternal Health and American Cultural Values*,
Global Maternal and Child Health, https://doi.org/10.1007/978-3-031-23969-4_3

(Margolis, 2000). Working mothers are persistently paid less than working women who are not mothers (Stoner, 2018).

Gradually, the childrearing model of motherhood shifted from sentimental (placing importance on emotional and moral qualities) toward intensive (with inherent expectations of mothers spending inordinate amounts of time, energy, and money) childrearing (Doyle, 2018; Gross, 2018; Hays, 1996). Contemporary motherhood in America is complicated by continued race and class inequities and implicit expectations that women live up to a blended ideal of motherhood requiring intensive childrearing while participating in the nation's workforce and sentimentally experiencing complete joy and fulfillment because they are mothers (Hays, 1996; Margolis, 2000; Regev, 2015; Vandenberg-Daves, 2014). A two-income family is the norm demanded by the post WWII consumer-driven society and intensive childrearing which entails time intensive and often expensive social requirement (e.g., ballet lessons, buying new soccer uniforms every season, volunteering in the classroom). The expectation of intensive childrearing is that mothers should and will meet every physical, emotional, and social need of the child.

However, in reality, intensive childrearing is often contradictory to the very participation in the formal workforce that it seems to demand (Hays, 1996; Margolis, 2000). Current polls indicate that American women continue to face pressure to practice intensive childrearing even though they are also spending more time in the labor force (Geiger et al., 2019). Today's working women face multiple conflicts related to motherhood.

Whether women are contemplating future pregnancy or are already mothers, employment is an important consideration in obtaining health insurance coverage. While public assistance is available and has been expanded for unemployed or very low-income pregnant women (e.g., Medicaid for pregnancy), health insurance coverage is generally tied to employment. Choice and perceived quality of healthcare are linked to private insurance (Bailey, 2022; Lyonette et al., 2011; Markus et al., 2017; Martinez-Hume et al., 2017). However, employer-provided private health insurance coverage is usually dependent on full-time work (Lyonette et al., 2011).

Neither paid nor unpaid family leave is adequate. Not only is the amount of time allotted for maternity and family leave variable, paid leave is not a guaranteed benefit of employment.

The USA, Marshall Islands, and Papua New Guinea are the only countries in the world that do not offer legal maternity leave. The Family and Medical Leave Act (FMLA) of 1993 is a federal law guaranteeing 12 weeks of unpaid leave; however, not all employees are eligible for FMLA benefits. In March 2020, just 20% of private sector workers in the USA had employer provided paid leave. Family leave varies by state and often stipulates that the mother expend all available vacation days or sick time accumulated first in order to qualify for family leave (Glynn, 2019; Jung, 2018; *Mom congress*, 2021).

Childcare is also part of the equation for women in the paid workforce. Does the pay she earns adequately offset the tangible and intangible expenses of childcare? In the early 1990s, 3% of childcare was provided by a nanny, au pair, or housekeeper, 47% by a family member, and 48% at a daycare (Hays, 1996). The quality of childcare available to mothers is primarily dependent on what they can afford to pay. Women in lower paying jobs or those working part-time often rely on informal childcare arrangements. (Lyonette et al., 2011). In 2012, 75.2% of mothers working full-time relied on family members for childcare at least part of the time. The yearly cost for infant care in a formal childcare center is more expensive than annual tuition at an average public university (Glynn, 2012). Public assistance, the child care credit, is limited and few eligible families receive it (Glynn, 2019). Child care remains a tremendous financial burden, significantly worsened by the COVID-19 pandemic. The USA has some of the most expensive childcare in the world (*Mom congress*, 2021). For many, childcare is simply unavailable. On average, it requires at least 10% of household income (Kolmar, 2021).

Despite the progress made toward work place equality since WWII, an ideological lag continues. While both parents are often participating in the paid workforce, mothers often come home to *second shift* responsibilities. These responsibilities include childcare during hours at home, primary caregiving responsibility for a sick child, and most household chores (Glynn, 2019; Hays, 1996).

Successful motherhood is a socially constructed concept. What constitutes successful motherhood the USA is the culturally accepted meaning derived from having a family, biological or adopted (Hays, 1996). When confronted with family dysfunction, mothers are frequently blamed and held accountable for the overall wellbeing of society. Yet, professional success often garners a woman greater status than culturally-defined successful motherhood. Women juggle multiple roles, including parenting, sometimes at the expense of the cultural role of motherhood (Hays, 1996; Kumar, 2020; Margolis, 2000; Vandenberg-Daves, 2014).

3.2 Experiences Across Life

3.2.1 Life Course Theory

One's life is influenced by the social determinants of health (SDoH); socioeconomic status and stability, access to education and healthcare, and the built environment and social context in which she lives (Healthy People, 2030; Jones et al., 2019; UNFPA, 2012; World Health Organization, 2018).

Life course theory (LCT) emerged as an interdisciplinary theory with roots in anthropology, demography, psychology, sociology, and history (Hutchison, 2011). It has been applied to health and health disparity research (Jones et al., 2019; Mortimer & Shanahan, 2006). LCT is a holistic framework that acknowledges the influences of a woman's entire life on her current health and well-being. Prior life experiences and her response to those experiences influence decision-making

The overarching premise of LCT involves the inseparability of body and mind (Black et al., 2009). Three key concepts explained in life course theory are the *trajectory of a person's life, transitions to new life experiences*, and *turning points*

(Hutchison, 2011). The trajectory of a person's life describes the long and stable patterns in life, typically education, career, and a life partner. Transitions to new life experiences include entering a new role, such as motherhood.

Transitions are distinct as a new role begins. Turning points represent abrupt, substantial, and lasting changes (e.g., severe maternal morbidity or a maternal near-miss).

These three key concepts are further developed utilizing five components: *context, developmental stage, timing, agency*, and *linked lives* (Black et al., 2009). The components are not mutually exclusive, but rather overlapping and complementary.

3.2.2   Context

Geographic location and the socio-historical significance of that location are major components of context. Context specifics, such as urban crowding or rural isolation, geopolitical events (e.g., Black Lives Matter movement), economic cycles (e.g., record high unemployment rates during the COVID-19 pandemic), and cultural values (e.g., self-reliance) shape individual behavior and decision-making (Alwin, 2012).

When a mother enjoys high social standing with access to resources, she is apt to have less stress and better health. Conversely, mothers with limited social standing and resources are more likely to be stressed. Without adequate resources to buffer negative life events, women are at risk for increased stress and depression. Mothers living in the context of systemic racial and gender discrimination are negatively impacted by chronic stress regardless of socioeconomics (Owens & Jackson, 2015).

Context is as nuanced and varied as communities are across the nation. Understanding context as an important element of life course is crucial to anticipating or mitigating risks which may affect maternal health. Context includes not only individual mothers, but the family and community (Cheng & Solomon, 2014), thus complementing the *linked lives* component of LCT.

3.2.3   Developmental Stage

In terms of reproductive health, developmental stages encompass preconception, prenatal, intrapartum, interconception, and postnatal periods. Developmental stages encompass milestones resulting from psychosocial processes and physical growth. Early life events, physical and mental health at earlier developmental stages, and environmental exposures at any point of the life influence risk and protective factors. Young girls are linked to their future as mothers.

Significant physiologic or psychosocial stressors experienced at any developmental stage can affect maternal health and their role as a mother (Allen et al., 2014; Halfon et al., 2014; Misra & Grason, 2006).

3.2.4 Timing

Health age must be considered in terms of chronological age, and age-related changes. A woman's perceptions of health age influences perceived deadlines for important transitions in life, such as when to become a mother. Positive influences in a woman's life have the potential to reduce risk factors and improve outcomes throughout all reproductive developmental stages. Managing exposures during the antenatal period has the potential to influence the live-long health of both mother and child.

Timing, perceived deadlines, and the flexibility of those deadlines vary individually. Large-scale changes affect entire populations and influence one's subjective experience of an altered life course (Alwin, 2012; Misra & Grason, 2006; Vandenberg-Daves, 2014). Sociocultural changes, influence women's perceptions of motherhood. For example, American women entering the work force during WWII, and the "modern age" of motherhood required mothers to be educated in "scientific" methods of childrearing. Large scale changes can influence individual women's timing for motherhood, as many highly educated, career-minded women choose to delay motherhood. The average age of first-time mothers in 1994 was 23 and had increased to age 26 by 2014 (Geiger et al., 2019). Career-focused women may not desire motherhood less than other women, but are willing to wait until they perceive the timing to be right, despite increased risks associated with advanced maternal age pregnancies and possible expense and effort required to preserve fertility or engage with assisted reproductive technology (Simoni et al., 2017).

3.2.5 Agency

Agency is personal control. Making plans, modifying expectations, and adapting to circumstances are all part of personal control. American women are active decision-makers within opportunities and constraints perceived. Their perceptions of their own levels of agency are influenced by self-efficacy, intellectual ability, having determination and self-control, a sense of personal accountability, and life context. Individuals who believe they can influence their own destiny may have an internal locus of control, whereas individuals with a fatalistic view that they are victims of circumstance may have an external locus of control. Perceptions of agency can either be protective or increase risk associated with motherhood across a woman's life course (Alwin, 2012; Mortimer & Shanahan, 2003). The following composite case study is an example of how LCT provides a framework understanding the influences that affect decision-making and maternal health outcomes. This story also exemplifies context, developmental stage, timing, agency and linked lives but in particular it highlights *agency*.

Box 3.1 Sara's Strength: A Life Course Story of Agency

A tiny agitated baby girl was abandoned in a neighborhood grocery store at about 4 months of age. She had no identification or clues as to her mother's identity or her family of origin. This baby could have faced potentially devastating social determinants. Instead, she was taken in by the grocer's family, named Sara, and raised by this large extended family. Given a home and identity of sorts, she had an informal last name as she was not adopted. At that time and place, stray children were often just absorbed into a family. There was hope that one day a mother might resurface. There were no Baby Moses or Safe Haven laws in place.

When I first met Sara, I realized that she was a feisty, determined young woman. She had musical talent and worked as a DJ. Her pregnancy was a surprise, but already she was beginning to cherish the baby. Sara had support from her coworkers and her childhood family, enabling her to have plans for her child's life. During the pregnancy, this young mother attended childbirth and breastfeeding classes, showed up for clinic visits, and bonded to her developing baby. Occasionally she shared her life—a thin veil between what is heavenly and what is truth. Pregnancy is often a time when the mind and heart receive great insights, when dreams are only a few degrees separated from reality. We talked about the essentials that she received as a child, building her sense of agency. Limited in resources, the grocer's family gave her attention, time, care, and love. We talked about the greatest blessing a child can have, being loved by a family committed to parenting and certainty. Visits often extended beyond the 20 allotted minutes, prompting the schedulers to put Sara at the end of the day, wise to the ways that healing takes time and attention.

Sara had dabbled some with drugs. At her first prenatal visit, she tested positive test for methamphetamine. Although not documented, Sara's biological family situation may have been like others—grandmothers active with alcohol abuse, mothers who abused cannabis, trickling down to the next generation abusing methamphetamine or opioids. However, during the pregnancy Sara became clean and sober, an accomplishment achieved across three months and motivated by her pregnancy. We would spend time discussing the balance of work and play, her relationship with the baby's father, and "life." As trust developed, we discussed the very real chance that Sara's baby might be the first baby born in three generations clean and sober. Eyes shifted up, a smile on her lips, good fetal heart reactivity, and the process unfolded. Sara loved her baby even before birth.

Labor was fun, at least for the providers and a friend from work and her "adopted" mother who raised her who sang to her and chanted "You can do it, Sara," In standing position, with full control and guided pushing, Sara birthed her perfect baby, bringing her little one to her breast for the first of many feedings. Success sprung up around every corner.

In the weeks and months that followed, I would see Sara walking around town, carrying her little one in a front pack, looking just as if her life as a mother could have been predicted but in fact was a miracle of childhood confidence building. Beginning life in desperate circumstances, Sara brought the gift of agency giving her baby a real chance.

This story challenges textbook explanations of maternal outcomes. It causes us to listen more deeply for tales of sacrifice, grace, and the value of linked lives embedded in the life course of mothers.

Personal communication, Martha Hoffman Goedert, PhD, CNM, May 13, (2022)

3.2.6 Linked Lives

Relationships and social ties link women's lives to those around them. Within this network of linked lives, any major changes affecting one member (marriage, death, job loss) has an effect on the rest of the members. Wellbeing within the network is generally promoted as members support each other and reinforce bonds. When tension occurs between an individual member's goals and the collective needs of the network, ties may be broken, causing deterioration of the network.

Life course theory views motherhood throughout the developmental stages. For example, a woman's access to health insurance and healthcare throughout her life, her health habits, risk factors, such as obesity or substance abuse, and development and management of noncommunicable chronic diseases such as gestational diabetes, affect her maternal health (Azenha et al., 2013; Graham et al., 2010; Jacob et al., 2020; McClain et al., 2019; Misra & Grason, 2006). One's sense of personal control in adulthood is associated with educational level (Mirowsky & Ross, 2007). Educational inequity affects health literacy and the knowledge base to make healthcare decisions (Azenha et al., 2013). Like the previous case study, the following composite case study exemplifies context, developmental stage, timing, agency and linked lives but in particular it highlights *linked lives*.

A healthy, young first-time mother faithfully attended her prenatal visits at a First Nations clinic that is a trusted haven by the community. Her pregnancy progressed normally and the baby's growth and development were perfect. All examinations, ultrasounds, and tests were normal. Eerily at each visit she voiced *knowing* that she would die in childbirth.

Concerned about this focus on death, the midwives assured her that she was healthy, listening as she shared her hopes and dreams for her child, and observing for communication cues and signs of mental illness. Throughout antenatal screening, the mother expressed fear of her controlling, rageful partner. She shared with her midwives her history of intimate partner abuse and the cyclic nature of this abuse in her relationship, even during pregnancy. Her 'third eye' inner voice expressed the knowing that she would die in childbirth, not at the hand of her abuser.

> **Box 3.2 Knowing: A Life Course Story of Linked Lives**
> The healthcare team carefully assessed her home situation, shared resources for her personal safety, offered guidance on the cycle of intimate partner violence and the dynamics of power and control, and assessed her mental health. She was counseled and offered assistance to relocate to a safer home environment with relatives. She resisted any changes and the team respected her autonomy, realizing that the nuances of her life were hers to share as she chose. She continued to express *knowing* that she would die in childbirth.
>
> During childbirth, this healthy young woman developed an amniotic fluid embolism. Rapid and heroic measures brought forth a wellborn baby but the mother did not survive. However, that is not the end of the story. All along, she said she *knew* she would die in childbirth. She told her family she wanted her cherished baby to be raised, safe and secure, in the matriarchal circle of the extended family. She perceived that if she lived, she would have no choice but to return to the abusive, toxic environment in the father's family. By her death, she culturally punted the care and raising of the child to the matriarchs on her side of the extended family.
>
> This story challenges textbook explanations of maternal outcomes. It causes us to listen more deeply for tales of sacrifice and grace and to appreciate the values of linked lives in the life course of mothers.
>
> Personal communication, Martha Hoffman Goedert, PhD, CNM, May 13, (2022)

3.3 American Cultural Values Shaping Motherhood

Women's lived experiences of motherhood may conflict with cultural representations of American motherhood (Doyle, 2018). Attitudes toward motherhood are, in part, shaped by cultural messages about gender, which has been slow to shift from patriarchal roots despite the feminist movement in the USA (Cruea, 2005). A mismatch persists between socially-constructed gender messages and what women experience (Gross, 2018).

While culture emphasizes the emotional satisfaction of becoming a mother, a woman's experience of becoming a mother may be fraught with physical, emotional, and mental pain and suffering (Gross, 2018). Since the 1800s, a mothering the USA has been characterized as a White middle-class married woman, which excludes other women from fully identifying with the American ideal of motherhood (Doyle, 2018; Williams, 2021). Women outside of this narrow parameter experience increased scrutiny of their role as mothers. For instance, women with disabilities may be discouraged from adopting, experience interference in maintaining custody of their children, or expected to prevent or terminate pregnancy. Strangers observing mothers with disabilities caring for their children often feel compelled to evaluate her worthiness or make well-intentioned comments belying their distrust of the woman's mothering ability (Taussig, 2021). Similarly, though cohabitating individuals having a child together outside of marriage has gained acceptance and in many places is the norm, stigma persists around single motherhood (Sawhill et al., 2010). Single mothers are viewed as creating fragile families requiring public assistance. They may be depicted as welfare queens (Aquilino, 1996; Cassese & Barnes, 2019). Societal support for public assistance is influenced by social class, gender, and ethnicity, which in turn shapes policy (Cassese & Barnes, 2019; Williams, 2021). Mothers requiring public assistance may be viewed as lacking the value of personal control and undeserving of assistance..

Women in perilous economic condition are often reluctant to become mothers. It is one way that some women choose to exercise control of their economic status, clearly demonstrated on survey research done in the early months of the COVID-19 pandemic (Cohen, 2021; Kahn et al., 2021). Declining fertility rates were linked to the 2008 financial recession and to the COVID-19 pandemic in birth rate in 2020, the largest drop in the USA since the early 1970s (Cohen, 2021; Hamilton et al., 2021).

However, not all women have full control of their own reproductive life. Reproductive coercion occurs for a variety of reasons, limiting women's choices (Grace et al., 2020).

Restrictive access to birth control and reproductive healthcare as well as cultural conflicts regarding women's reproductive choices further impact the choice to be a mother in America. "In reality, once a woman in America today becomes a mother, our society transports her back in time, to the 1950s. In an instant, generations of sexist ideas and structure descend back upon her" (Tenety, 2021, para. 3). Women consider the *motherhood penalty* in their reproductive decision-making. The employed mothers' penalty consists of inequality in hiring, advancement, pay, and training/career opportunities (Kumar, 2020). The COVID-19 pandemic has highlighted the need for increased investment in supports for employed mothers. However, legislation has focused on competing business interests (Roosevelt, 2021; Williams, 2021). American cultural values dichotomize the roles of mother and employee (McQuillan et al., 2008). Yet, both identities reflect the intersectional reality of the life course for many American women.

3.4 Summary

This chapter examines how patterns of decision-making, grounded in core American cultural values, have profoundly influenced the lived experiences and health outcomes of mothers. Maternal health continues to be subsumed by infant outcomes. Advocacy for policies to promote maternal health (such as maternity leave) are often driven by pressure to decrease untoward infant outcomes related to preterm birth and other factors (Kenner et al., 2018; Misra & Grason, 2006).American healthcare policies are data driven. However, behind the measures of maternal health are cultural values that influence decision-making about funding priorities (Brunson & Suh, 2020; Misra & Grason, 2006).

References

Allen, D., Feinberg, E., & Mitchell, H. (2014). Bringing life course home: A pilot to reduce pregnancy risk through housing access and family support. *Maternal and Child Health Journal, 18*(2), 405–412.

Alwin, D. F. (2012). Integrating varieties of life course concepts. *The Journals of Gerontology, 67*(2), 206–220.

Aquilino, W. S. (1996). The life course of children born to unmarried mothers: Childhood living arrangements and young adult outcomes. *Journal of Marriage and the Family*, 293–310.

Azenha, G. S., Parsons-Perez, C., Goltz, S., Bhadelia, A., Durstine, A., Knaul, F., Torode, J., Starrs, A., McGuire, H., & Kidwell, J. D. (2013). Recommendations towards an integrated, life-course approach to women's health in the post-2015 agenda. *Bulletin of the World Health Organization, 91*, 704–706.

Bailey, V. (2022). HRSA expands preventive care coverage under ACA for women, children. *Health Payer Intelligence*. Retrieved January 14, 2022, from https://healthpayerintelligence.com/news/hrsa-expands-preventive-care-coverage-under-aca-for-women-children

Black, B. P., Holditch-Davis, D., & Miles, M. S. (2009). Life course theory as a framework to examine becoming a mother of a medically fragile preterm infant. *Research in Nursing & Health, 32*(1), 38–49.

Brunson, J., & Suh, S. (2020). Behind the measures of maternal and reproductive health: Ethnographic accounts of inventory and intervention. *Social Science & Medicine, 254*, 112730.

Cassese, E. C., & Barnes, T. D. (2019). Intersectional motherhood: Investigating public support for child care subsidies. *Politics, Groups, and Identities, 7*(4), 775–793.

Cheng, T. L., & Solomon, B. S. (2014). Translating life course theory to clinical practice to address health disparities. *Maternal and Child Health Journal, 18*(2), 389–395.

Cohen, P. N. (2021). Disrupted family plans and exacerbated inequalities associated with COVID-19 pandemic. *JAMA Network Open, 4*(9), e2124399–e2124399.

Cruea, S. M. (2005). Changing ideals of womanhood during the nineteenth-century woman movement. *ATQ, 19*(3), 187.

Doyle, N. (2018). *Maternal bodies: Redefining motherhood in early America*. The University of North Carolina Press.

Geiger, A. W., Livingston, G., & Bialik, K. (2019). *6 facts about U.S* (moms). Numbers. https://www.pewresearch.org/fact-tank/2019/05/08/facts-about-u-s-mothers/

Glynn, S. J. (2012). *Families need more help to care for their children* (child care fact sheet, issue). https://www.americanprogress.org/article/fact-sheet-child-care/

Glynn, S. J. (2019). *Breadwinning mothers continue to be the U.S. norm.* https://www.american-progress.org/article/breadwinning-mothers-continue-u-s-norm/

Grace, K. T., Alexander, K. A., Jeffers, N. K., Miller, E., Decker, M. R., Campbell, J., & Glass, N. (2020). Experiences of reproductive coercion among Latina women and strategies for minimizing harm: "the path makes us strong". *Journal of Midwifery & Women's Health, 65*(2), 248–256.

Graham, H., Hawkins, S. S., & Law, C. (2010). Lifecourse influences on women's smoking before, during and after pregnancy. *Social Science & Medicine, 70*(4), 582–587.

Gross, J. L. (2018). Maternal bodies: Redefining motherhood in early America. *Civil War Book Review, 20*(4), 27.

Halfon, N., Larson, K., Lu, M., Tullis, E., & Russ, S. (2014). Lifecourse health development: Past, present and future. *Maternal and Child Health Journal, 18*(2), 344–365.

Hamilton, B. E., Martin, J. A., & Osterman, M. J. (2021). *Births: Provisional data for* 2020. Vital statistics rapid release, National Vital Statistics System. NCHS Report No. 012.

Hays, S. (1996). *The cultural contradictions of motherhood. Yale University Press. Healthy People 2030, U.S.* Department of Health and Human Services. https://health.gov/healthypeople/objectives-and-data/social-determinants-health

Hutchison, E. D. (2011). *Life course theory.* Encyclopedia of Adolescence.

Jacob, C. M., Briana, D. D., Di Renzo, G. C., Modi, N., Bustreo, F., Conti, G., Malamitsi-Puchner, A., & Hanson, M. (2020). Building resilient societies after COVID-19: the case for investing in maternal, neonatal, and child health. *The Lancet Public Health.* https://doi.org/10.1016/S2468-2667(20)30200-0

Jones, N. L., Gilman, S. E., Cheng, T. L., Drury, S. S., Hill, C. V., & Geronimus, A. T. (2019). Life course approaches to the causes of health disparities. *American Journal of Public Health, 109*(S1), S48–S55.

Jung, H. (2018). *Policy at a glance: State & federal policies for maternity leave.* Loma Linda University Health Institute for Health Policy and Leadership.

Kahn, L. G., Trasande, L., Liu, M., Mehta-Lee, S. S., Brubaker, S. G., & Jacobson, M. H. (2021). Factors associated with changes in pregnancy intention among women who were mothers of young children in new York City following the COVID-19 outbreak. *JAMA Network Open, 4*(9), e2124273–e2124273.

Kenner, C., Ashford, K., Badr, L. K., Black, B., Bloch, J., Mainous, R., McGrath, J., Premji, S., Sinclair, S., & Terhaar, M. (2018). American Academy of Nursing on policy: Reducing preterm births in the United States: Maternal infant health, child, adolescent and family, and women's health expert panels (August 13, 2018). *Nursing Outlook, 66*, 499.

Kolmar, C. (2021). *US child care availability statistics (childcare availability statistics).* Issue. Z. Research. https://www.zippia.com/advice/us-child-care-availability-statistics/

Kumar, S. (2020). The motherhood penalty: Not so Black and white. *Electronic Thesis and Dissertation Repository, 7157.* https://ir.lib.uwo.ca/etd/7157

Lyonette, C., Kaufman, G., & Crompton, R. (2011). 'We both need to work' maternal employment, childcare and health care in Britain and the USA. *Work, Employment and Society, 25*(1), 34–50.

Margolis, M. L. (2000). *True to her nature: Changing advice to American women.* Waveland Press.

Markus, A. R., Krohe, S., Garro, N., Gerstein, M., & Pellegrini, C. (2017). Examining the association between Medicaid coverage and preterm births using 2010–2013 National Vital Statistics Birth Data. *Journal of Children and Poverty, 23*(1), 79–94.

Martinez-Hume, A. C., Baker, A. M., Bell, H. S., Montemayor, I., Elwell, K., & Hunt, L. M. (2017). "They treat you a different way:" public insurance, stigma, and the challenge to quality health care. *Culture, Medicine, and Psychiatry, 41*(1), 161–180.

McClain, A. C., Dickin, K. L., & Dollahite, J. (2019). Life course influences on food provisioning among low-income, Mexican-born mothers with young children at risk of food insecurity. *Appetite, 132*, 8–17.

McQuillan, J., Greil, A. L., Shreffler, K. M., & Tichenor, V. (2008). The importance of motherhood among women in the contemporary United States. *Gender & Society, 22*(4), 477–496.

Mirowsky, J., & Ross, C. E. (2007). Life course trajectories of perceived control and their relationship to education. *American Journal of Sociology, 112*(5), 1339–1382.

Misra, D. P., & Grason, H. (2006). Achieving safe motherhood: Applying a life course and multiple determinants perinatal health framework in public health. *Women's Health Issues, 16*(4), 159–175.

Mom congress. (2021). Mom Congress. https://www.mom-congress.com/our-issues?gclid=Cj0KCQjw5auGBhDEARIsAFyNm9GQfRK_hwVMbISVRZflGTCSKo7SaAVZk8CIc_yKWQncL9jp_oaqlisaAqyMEALw_wcB

Mortimer, J. T., & Shanahan, M. (2003). *Handbook of the life course (handbooks of sociology and social research).* Kluwer Academic.

Mortimer, J. T., & Shanahan, M. J. (2006). *Handbook of the life course.* Springer.

Owens, T. C., & Jackson, F. M. (2015). Examining life-course socioeconomic position, contextualized stress, and depression among well-educated African-American pregnant women. *Women's Health Issues, 25*(4), 382–389.

Regev, M. (2015). The myth of motherhood: The way unrealistic social expectations of mothers shape their experience. *Dr. Regev.* https://drregev.com/blog/the-myth-of-motherhood-the-way-unrealistic-social-expectations-of-mothers-shape-their-experience/

Roosevelt, M. (2021). More workplace protections in 2022. *Los Angeles Times, 1.*

Sawhill, I., Thomas, A., & Monea, E. (2010). An ounce of prevention: Policy prescriptions to reduce the prevalence of fragile families. *The Future of Children, 20*, 133–155.

Simoni, M. K., Mu, L., & Collins, S. C. (2017). Women's career priority is associated with attitudes towards family planning and ethical acceptance of reproductive technologies. *Human Reproduction, 32*(10), 2069–2075.

Stoner, R. (2018). How to make motherhood easier in America. *Pacific Standard.* https://psmag.com/economics/how-to-make-motherhood-easier-in-america.

Taussig, R. (2021). Baby steps: Learning to parent in public after a year in our cozy cave. *Time, 4.* https://time.com/5958537/pandemic-baby-disabled-mom-rebekah-taussig/

Tenety, E. (2021). It's 2021, but for American mothers, it's still the 1950s. *Motherly.* https://www.mother.ly/life/for-american-mothers-its-1950s/

UNFPA. (2012). *Rich mother, poor mother: The social determinants of maternal death and disability.* UNFPA. https://www.unfpa.org/resources/social-determinants-maternal-death-and-disability.

Vandenberg-Daves, J. (2014). *Modern motherhood: An American history.* Rutgers University Press.

Williams, H. H. (2021). Just mothering: Amy Coney Barrett and the racial politics of American motherhood. *Laws, 10*(2), 36.

World Health Organization. (2018). *Maternal and newborn health: Life-course approach.* WHO. http://www.euro.who.int/en/health-topics/Life-stages/maternal- and-newborn-health/maternal-and-newborn-health

Chapter 4
Fertility and Reproductive Health

Lisa R. Roberts

4.1 Fertility and Reproductive Health in the USA

Despite prior research indicating that motherhood is highly valued and desired by most American women, fertility rates have drastically decreased (Arnett, 1998; Hamilton et al., 2021; McQuillan et al., 2008). In 1950, the total fertility rate was 3.09. By 1980, it had decreased to 1.80, and in 2019, it was 1.75 (GBD Collaborators & Ärnlöv, 2020). In 2020, births in the USA dropped still further, attributing to the COVID-19 pandemic altering fertility intentions (Cohen, 2021). The downward trend in fertility is closely tied to fertility intentions, as the 2019 contraception prevalence rate in the USA of 73.9% indicates that most women have access to contraception (CIA, 2022), although there are still barriers to reproductive health.

A woman's fertility intentions (number and spacing of children desired) vary over the course of her life and also vary greatly among women. Factors influencing fertility intentions include reproductive health, prior birth experiences, religiosity, social determinants of health (SDoH) such as education and socioeconomic status, and cultural factors such as social pressure to conform to pronatalist messages (*motherhood mandate*), and gender attitudes. The perceived importance of motherhood and the importance of building a family impacts fertility intentions and life course (Berrington & Pattaro, 2014; Buhr & Huinink, 2014; Gemmill, 2019; Hayford, 2009; Kuhnt et al., 2021; McQuillan et al., 2015). These factors reflect cultural values that influence a woman's decisions about her fertility.

L. R. Roberts (✉)
Loma Linda University, Loma Linda, CA, USA

© The Author(s), under exclusive license to Springer Nature Switzerland AG 2023   43
B. A. Anderson, L. R. Roberts (eds.), *Maternal Health and American Cultural Values*,
Global Maternal and Child Health, https://doi.org/10.1007/978-3-031-23969-4_4

4.2 Influence of American Cultural Values

Practicality is an American cultural value that places high value on efficiency, cost-effectiveness, and managing resources. Healthcare interventions and technology used in reproductive healthcare are highly regarded. The American tendency to be action oriented also comes into play, creating tension between expectant management and rapid intervention at the time of childbirth. These cultural values influence decisions about fertility and reproductive health from the individual to the national policy level. Women deciding *if* and *when* to have children face expectations to conform to implicit maternal behaviors and take action to ensure specific outcomes. In our action-oriented society, practical solutions are often prioritized over lengthy contemplation of causes of inequity. Cost-based policy decisions may create barriers to reproductive care, especially with infertility, and further drive healthcare disparities.

4.2.1 Women of Diverse Backgrounds

Women of color, adolescent or young adult aged women, LGBTQ+, women with disabilities, and those living in rural areas are more likely to face barriers to reproductive care. Barriers include maternal healthcare deserts, variance in quality and availability of care, gaps in provider knowledge about the needs and preferences of various women, and discrimination. Reproductive healthcare policies and insurance coverage that have not kept pace with changes in society, medical advances, and healthcare workforce shortages (Anderson & Roberts, 2019; Mazur et al., 2018; Moseson et al., 2020; Prather et al., 2018; Taouk et al., 2018; Wingo et al., 2018). Women of diverse groups are also more likely to have had negative prior birth experiences despite global initiatives to provide safe, respectful maternal care (United Nations, 2019).

4.2.2 Negative Birth Experience

Negative birth experiences have been estimated to occur in 10% to 27% of births in the USA. These experiences impact postpartum adjustment and future fertility intentions. Negative experiences include power imbalances, discrimination, disrespectful treatment by healthcare providers, rude behavior, inattention, withholding information, and judgmental, disapproving comments. These experiences may result in loss of autonomy and coercion (Attanasio et al., 2021; Edmonds et al., 2021; Glazer et al., 2021; Preis et al., 2020; Roth et al., 2014; United Nations, 2019; Vedam et al., 2019; Villines, 2019). American mothers, particularly those representing diverse groups, may be subject to societal messages that contribute to loss of autonomy and may be tantamount to victim blaming (Crawford, 1977).

All mothers deserve to be treated with respect during childbearing. Respectful maternity care (RMC) is a United Nations initiative intended to promote inclusive, nondiscriminatory, affordable, accessible, and acceptable care. Acceptability of care requires that the recipient feels safe and secure physically and psychologically. It ensures care provided with dignity, compassion, and privacy. It is more than the absence of mistreatment. Guided by principles of essential human rights, it is hampered by inconsistently defined terms, the lack of objective measures, varying policies, and unreliable operationalization (Beecher et al., 2021; Jolivet et al., 2021; Lalonde et al., 2019; United Nations, 2019). The perception of disrespectful care may influence fertility intentions.

4.2.3 Expectations of Family Structure

Religious beliefs are often associated with increased fertility intentions and valuing large families. Pronatalist messaging may have greater influence than the norm of the two-child family. Religiosity and pronatal messaging are closely tied to traditional gender attitudes influencing fertility intentions. Traditional gender attitudes are supported by the tenet that women should be the primary caretakers of home and children. Among fundamentalist groups, these factors are even more pronounced. Children may be viewed as a source of social cohesion and validation of community gender roles (Hayford, 2009; Margolis, 2019; McQuillan et al., 2015; Pearce, 2002).

Family structure affects the amount of time parents spend in caring for children. While social norms may endorse an *ideal* family structure consisting of highly available mother, a wage-earning father, and two children, the reality is often different. Family structures are often diverse and complex, not fitting with this model. The prevailing wisdom is that the highly available mother fits the pattern of *intensive mothering* described in Chap. 3, including the amount of time spent in caring for children. However, in the USA, single parents often spend more time with their children than cohabitating or married parents, even though single parents also work more and experience greater income inequality compared to dual-parent families. Children raised in single-parent households are also more likely to earn lower incomes as adults (Bloome, 2017; Hays, 1996; Kalenkoski et al., 2007; Kennedy & Fitch, 2012; Krueger et al., 2015). Despite the two-child norm as the *ideal* family structure in American culture, in reality it may not be compatible with the American cultural value of practicality and action-orientation. American women are not inclined to leave motherhood up to destiny.

4.3 Distress and Ambivalence about Motherhood

Women who do not desire children may experience *othering*. Voluntary childlessness (described as child-free) often results in stigma, marginalization, and oppression. Despite declining fertility rates, women without fertility intentions are still considered the exception to the rule, and are often hesitant to express their ambivalence toward motherhood, due to the very real possibility of marginalization. The sociopolitical narrative of the *motherhood mandate* results in women choosing to remain childless to be viewed as pitiable, selfish, or menacing. In the context of declining fertility, pronatal views and family friendly policies may even be encouraged as a way to increase the fertility rate and sustain the nation's workforce. Political rhetoric consistently refers to the well-being of mothers and families, not childless women, and in doing so creates *othering* and loss of autonomy (Cain, 2022; Gotlib, 2016).

Despite overt pronatalist messaging, there are strong implicit messages that do not support motherhood. Family-leave policies (both paid and unpaid) are inadequate, mothers are often denied job promotion or unequally compensated by employers, and childcare, generally not subsidized, is inordinately expensive. Some careers or life circumstances are incompatible with having children, and thus are responsible for women choosing to remain childless. Some women delay childbearing in pursuit of higher education, career, or other goals until they are no longer interested in motherhood, or childlessness becomes an outcome rather than an active choice. In short, sociopolitical, economic, and personal circumstances are not always conducive to motherhood, despite the *motherhood mandate* (Cain, 2022; Gemmill, 2019; Gotlib, 2016; Hays, 1996; Jung, 2018; Kolmar, 2021).

4.4 Infertility

Women who do not *choose* to be childless, but rather have infertility issues, experience disappointment, pain and suffering, grief, and altered life plans. A recent systematic review found that only half of women experiencing infertility pursue treatment (Cebert-Gaitors et al., 2021). Women experiencing infertility often have greater fertility intention than women without fertility issues. Even when infertility treatment is successful, delays in experiencing childbearing, grueling treatment regimens, decreased number of desired children, and emotional challenges are often significant (Marshall & Raynor, 2014; Shreffler et al., 2016).

The diagnostic process for infertility fills couples with self-doubt, fears, and stress. Procreation is no longer an intimate, personal affair. Failing to conceive within an expected timeframe, couples may be subject to social speculation, overt criticism, and well-meaning, often intrusive comments and suggestions. Once the decision is made to seek medical advice, both the woman and her male partner are required to answer often-overwhelming personal questions in identifying potential causes of the elusive embryo. For both the woman and her male partner, the process includes physical examination, genetic testing, blood tests, imaging, and hormonal tracking. Seeking treatment is more likely when fertility intention is high, both partners have high health literacy and desire a child, and there is family and community support (Cebert-Gaitors et al., 2021; Marshall & Raynor, 2014).

4.4.1 Assisted Reproductive Technology

Allopathic treatment for women with infertility currently includes ovarian stimulation with medications to regulate or induce ovulation, intrauterine insemination with either the partner's healthy sperm or donor sperm, surgery to correct physical impediments such as scar tissue or fibroids, or assisted reproductive technology (ART). ART is an overarching term for fertility treatment which involves managing egg and sperm through various methods, including the use of donor eggs, sperm, or embryos, and surrogacy. While ART is a means of attaining a desired pregnancy, it is not necessarily blissful. A recent systematic review indicated that women who are pregnant by ART experience feelings of uncertainty and ambivalence, bonding and development of maternal identity may be delayed, and the woman's social context and relationships are often altered (Maehara et al., 2022).

In vitro fertilization (IVF) is the most commonly used ART method. IVF requires the stimulation and retrieval of multiple eggs, fertilizing them with carefully prepared sperm in a petri dish, and then implanting the resulting embryos in the uterus several days after fertilization. IVF is common now and generally well accepted by society, but for the couple undergoing treatment, it may not feel commonplace at all. Treatment may result in complications such as bleeding or infection, ovarian hyperstimulation syndrome. Multiple pregnancy is more likely to occur with IVF (Burfoot & Güngör, 2022; Gawel, 2022; Marshall & Raynor, 2014). IVF resulting in a high number of viable embryos draws public scrutiny and highlights American cultural values of practicality and action-orientation.

A highly controversial example is *Octomom,* who conceived through IVF and gave birth to octuplets. Social outrage ensued regarding her fitness as a mother (a single, non-White woman who already had six children under eight years of age, and lived with her parents, supporting herself on worker's compensation and disability benefits), triggered professional and legislative decision-making. Questions arose around her mental health status and ability to parent, and the medical ethics of implanting so many embryos. These questions prompted regulation of *who* can conduct ART and *what* may be done via ART. Disadvantages of professional regulation include the possibility of discrimination favoring majority values (such as married heterosexual couples rather than single people or homosexuals). Regardless of *Octomom's* social and economic status, multiple births carry increased risk for both mother and babies, particularly at such a high number of multiples. Advantages of legislative decision-making include transparency and equal application the law, although state-to-state variances persist, including regulations about compensation for surrogacy. The fertility industry in the USA has recruited diverse donors, so as to attract national and international clients with the message that complex and often socially controversial procedures (e.g., surrogacy for male homosexual couples) are available (Jacobson, 2020; Perkins et al., 2018; Rao, 2015). Practicality and action-orientation influence norms and policy as families take action to fulfill their fertility intentions.

4.4.2 Social Response to Infertility

Despite the advances made in the diagnosis and treatment of infertility, and the acceptance of these modalities within American society, socioeconomic and racial disparity in access persists. Although online fertility consultations and self-collection of reproductive hormones specimens are available, treatment costs are prohibitive and insurance coverage is limited. Discrimination and commercial interests influence access in the USA (Burfoot & Güngör, 2022; Cebert-Gaitors et al., 2021; Gawel, 2022; Worthington et al., 2020). An example is freezing eggs. Some women choose to freeze their eggs while pursuing higher education or careers, or when undergoing treatment of health issues that would render them infertile. Egg freezing effectively preserves fertility intentions while delaying actual childbearing until perceived life conditions are deemed more ideal for family building (Baldwin et al., 2019; Gawel, 2022). Whether ART is chosen to delay or preserve fertility, or in the context of infertility, these are examples of practicality and action-orientation as American social values. As a woman enters the world of ART, she begins to experience the realities of *intensive mothering*. Her life now revolves around expert medical guidance and monitoring, and expenditure of personal time and resources. She now becomes accountable for deliberative actions to optimize the wellbeing of her offspring (Faircloth & Gürtin, 2018).

4.5 Family Building Alternatives

Surrogacy and adoption are options for building a family when motherhood is desired. Some women have economic restraints or are ineligible for IVF/ART, or have experienced a lack of success with treatments. They may consider surrogacy or adoption as secondary or alternative options. Others may consider surrogacy or adoption their first choice for family building.

When ART involves surrogacy, the gestational carrier is a woman who is genetically unrelated to the baby. Using gestational carriers may be desired due to a higher success rate than other IVF procedures, though the risk of multiple births remains a concern. Women choosing motherhood through surrogacy must be prepared to contend with the unpredictability of this and other complications, such as the possibility of a custody battle—whether the gestational surrogate acted altruistically, or was compensated (Perkins et al., 2018; Quinn, 2018; Tsai et al., 2020). While ART may be viewed as an alternative to adoption, adoption may be the preferred choice for some women.

Adoption in the USA may be pursued through the state-regulated program, *fost-adopt,* private informal arrangements, or legally recognized domestic or international adoption. Women may choose motherhood through any or all of these avenues, whether infertility is a factor or not. Motherhood can be created or expanded through adoption, rather than having any or increasing the number of biological children. Altruism, familiarity with the adoption process, or prior connection with a particular child are often motivating factors for adoption. Similarly, single or lesbian women may be motivated to adopt as the most practical way to achieve motherhood.

However, the American cultural context may present barriers. The USA is a racially stratified society with concerns about interethnic adoption. Furthermore, costs and lengthy waits, fear of losing custody, contact with the biological parents required, and fear of receiving an unhealthy or defective child may cause hesitation (Khanna & Killian, 2015; Malm & Welti, 2010). The American cultural values of practicality and action-orientation help many American women to overcome these barriers to motherhood.

4.6 Summary

The path to motherhood among American women may be as varied as the women themselves. The *motherhood mandate* affects women differently depending on their desire for or ambiguity toward motherhood. A woman's ability to act on her choices is based upon a culture that supports practicality and action-orientation. Assuming the role of motherhood and coherence with the *motherhood mandate* is usually a choice within the American culture.

References

Anderson, B. A., & Roberts, L. R. (Eds.). (2019). *The maternal health crisis in America: Nursing implications for advocacy and practice.* Springer.

Arnett, J. J. (1998). Learning to stand alone: The contemporary American transition to adulthood in cultural and historical context. *Human Development, 41*(5–6), 295–315.

Attanasio, L. B., Ranchoff, B. L., & Geissler, K. H. (2021). Perceived discrimination during the childbirth hospitalization and postpartum visit attendance and content: Evidence from the listening to mothers in California survey. *PLoS One, 16*(6), e0253055.

Baldwin, K., Culley, L., Hudson, N., & Mitchell, H. (2019). Running out of time: Exploring women's motivations for social egg freezing. *Journal of Psychosomatic Obstetrics and Gynecology, 40*(2), 166–173.

Beecher, C., Greene, R., O'Dwyer, L., Ryan, E., White, M., Beattie, M., & Devane, D. (2021). Measuring women's experiences of maternity care: A systematic review of self-report survey instruments. *Women and Birth, 34*(3), 231–241.

Berrington, A., & Pattaro, S. (2014). Educational differences in fertility desires, intentions and behaviour: A life course perspective. *Advances in Life Course Research, 21*, 10–27.

Bloome, D. (2017). Childhood family structure and intergenerational income mobility in the United States. *Demography, 54*(2), 541–569.

Buhr, P., & Huinink, J. (2014). Fertility analysis from a life course perspective. *Demographic Research, 30*, 1293–1326. https://doi.org/10.4054/DemRes.2014.30.45

Burfoot, A., & Güngör, D. (2022). *Women and reproductive technologies: The socio-economic development of technologies changing the world.* Routledge. https://doi.org/10.4324/9780429467646

Cain, A. (2022). A film feeds a hunger for stories on the ambivalence of motherhood. *Los Angeles Times.* Section A16, Sunday, Jan. 23, 2022 edition.

Cebert-Gaitors, M., Abdelnalbi, S., Mantell, E., Woodward, A., Gonzalez-Guarda, R., & Stevenson, E. L. (2021). Multidimensional barriers and facilitators to treatment seeking for infertility among women in the United States: A systemic review. *F&S Reviews, 3*(1), 76–89. https://doi.org/10.1016/j.xfnr.2021.10.001

CIA. (2022). *The world factbook: United States.* Central Intelligence Agency. Retrieved June 2, 2022 from https://www.cia.gov/the-world-factbook/countries/united-states/#people-and-society

Cohen, P. N. (2021). Disrupted family plans and exacerbated inequalities associated with COVID-19 pandemic. *JAMA Network Open, 4*(9), e2124399–e2124399.

Crawford, R. (1977). You are dangerous to your health: The ideology and politics of victim blaming. *International Journal of Health Services, 7*(4), 663–680.

Edmonds, J. K., Declercq, E., & Sakala, C. (2021). Women's childbirth experiences: A content analysis from the listening to mothers in California survey. *Birth, 00*, 1–9. https://doi.org/10.1111/birt.12531

Faircloth, C., & Gürtin, Z. B. (2018). Fertile connections: Thinking across assisted reproductive technologies and parenting culture studies. *Sociology, 52*(5), 983–1000.

Gawel, R. (2022). IVF treatment evolves to 'open up doors' for more diverse patient population. *Women's Health & OB/GYN.*. https://www.healio.com/news/womens-health-ob-gyn/20220209/ivf-treatment-evolves-to-open-up-doors-for-more-diverse-patient-population

GBD Collaborators, & Ärnlöv, J. (2020). Global age-sex-specific fertility, mortality, healthy life expectancy (HALE), and population estimates in 204 countries and territories, 1950–2019: A comprehensive demographic analysis for the global burden of disease study 2019. *The Lancet, 396*(10258), 1160–1203.

Gemmill, A. (2019). From some to none? Fertility expectation dynamics of permanently childless women. *Demography, 56*(1), 129–149.

Glazer, K. B., Sofaer, S., Balbierz, A., Wang, E., & Howell, E. A. (2021). Perinatal care experiences among racially and ethnically diverse mothers whose infants required a NICU stay. *Journal of Perinatology, 41*(3), 413–421.

Gotlib, A. (2016). "But you would be the best mother": Unwomen, counterstories, and the motherhood mandate. *Journal of Bioethical Inquiry, 13*(2), 327–347.

Hamilton, B. E., Martin, J. A., & Osterman, M. J. (2021). *Births: Provisional data for 2020.* Vital statistics rapid release (NCHS report no. 012).

Hayford, S. R. (2009). The evolution of fertility expectations over the life course. *Demography, 46*(4), 765–783.

Hays, S. (1996). *The cultural contradictions of motherhood.* Yale University Press.

Jacobson, H. (2020). Cross-border reproductive care in the USA: Who comes, why do they come, what do they purchase? *Reproductive Biomedicine & Society Online, 11*, 42–47. https://doi.org/10.1016/j.rbms.2020.09.003

Jolivet, R. R., Gausman, J., Kapoor, N., Langer, A., Sharma, J., & Semrau, K. E. (2021). Operationalizing respectful maternity care at the healthcare provider level: A systematic scoping review. *Reproductive Health, 18*(1), 1–15. https://doi.org/10.1186/s12978-021-01241-5

Jung, H. (2018). *Policy at a glance: State & federal policies for maternity leave.* Loma Linda University Health. https://ihpl.llu.edu/sites/ihpl.llu.edu/files/docs/Policy-At-A-Glance/september_2018_maternalleave.pdf

Kalenkoski, C. M., Ribar, D. C., & Stratton, L. S. (2007). The effect of family structure on parents' child care time in the United States and the United Kingdom. *Review of Economics of the Household, 5*(4), 353–384.

Kennedy, S., & Fitch, C. A. (2012). Measuring cohabitation and family structure in the United States: Assessing the impact of new data from the current population survey. *Demography, 49*(4), 1479–1498.

Khanna, N., & Killian, C. (2015). "We didn't even think about adopting domestically" the role of race and other factors in shaping parents' decisions to adopt abroad. *Sociological Perspectives, 58*(4), 570–594.

Kolmar, C. (2021). *US child care availability statistics.* Childcare availability statistics, Zippia Research. https://www.zippia.com/advice/us-child-care-availability-statistics/

Krueger, P. M., Jutte, D. P., Franzini, L., Elo, I., & Hayward, M. D. (2015). Family structure and multiple domains of child Well-being in the United States: A cross-sectional study. *Population Health Metrics, 13*(1), 1–11.

Kuhnt, A.-K., Minkus, L., & Buhr, P. (2021). Uncertainty in fertility intentions from a life course perspective: Which life course markers matter? *Journal of Family Research, 33*(1), 184–208.

Lalonde, A., Herschderfer, K., Pascali-Bonaro, D., Hanson, C., Fuchtner, C., & Visser, G. H. (2019). The international childbirth initiative: 12 steps to safe and respectful MotherBaby–family maternity care. *International Journal of Gynecology & Obstetrics, 146*(1), 65–73.

Maehara, K., Iwata, H., Kimura, K., & Mori, E. (2022). Experiences of transition to motherhood among pregnant women following assisted reproductive technology: A qualitative systematic review. *JBI Evidence Synthesis, 20*(3), 725–760. https://doi.org/10.11124/jbies-20-00545

Malm, K., & Welti, K. (2010). Exploring motivations to adopt. *Adoption Quarterly, 13*(3–4), 185–208.

Margolis, M. L. (2019). *Women in fundamentalism: Modesty, marriage, and motherhood.* Rowman & Littlefield.

Marshall, J., & Raynor, M. (Eds.). (2014). *Myles textbook for midwives* (16th ed.). Elsevier.

Mazur, A., Brindis, C. D., & Decker, M. J. (2018). Assessing youth-friendly sexual and reproductive health services: A systematic review. *BMC Health Services Research, 18*(1), 1–12.

McQuillan, J., Greil, A. L., Shreffler, K. M., & Bedrous, A. V. (2015). The importance of motherhood and fertility intentions among US women. *Sociological Perspectives, 58*(1), 20–35.

McQuillan, J., Greil, A. L., Shreffler, K. M., & Tichenor, V. (2008). The importance of motherhood among women in the contemporary United States. *Gender & Society, 22*(4), 477–496.

Moseson, H., Zazanis, N., Goldberg, E., Fix, L., Durden, M., Stoeffler, A., Hastings, J., Cudlitz, L., Lesser-Lee, B., & Letcher, L. (2020). The imperative for transgender and gender nonbinary inclusion: Beyond women's health. *Obstetrics and Gynecology, 135*(5), 1059.

Pearce, L. D. (2002). The influence of early life course religious exposure on young adults' dispositions toward childbearing. *Journal for the Scientific Study of Religion, 41*(2), 325–340.

Perkins, K. M., Boulet, S. L., Levine, A. D., Jamieson, D. J., & Kissin, D. M. (2018). Differences in the utilization of gestational surrogacy between states in the US. *Reproductive Biomedicine & Society Online, 5*, 1–4. https://doi.org/10.1016/j.rbms.2017.08.002

Prather, C., Fuller, T. R., Jeffries, W. L., IV, Marshall, K. J., Howell, A. V., Belyue-Umole, A., & King, W. (2018). Racism, African American women, and their sexual and reproductive health: A review of historical and contemporary evidence and implications for health equity. *Health equity, 2*(1), 249–259.

Preis, H., Tovim, S., Mor, P., Grisaru-Granovsky, S., Samueloff, A., & Benyamini, Y. (2020). Fertility intentions and the way they change following birth-a prospective longitudinal study. *BMC Pregnancy and Childbirth, 20*(1), 1–11.

Quinn, D. (2018). Her belly, their baby: A contract solution for surrogacy agreements. *JL & Pol'y, 26*(2), 805–846.

Rao, R. (2015). How (not) to regulate assisted reproductive technology: Lessons from octomom. *Fam. LQ, 49*(1), 135–147.

Roth, L. M., Heidbreder, N., Henley, M. M., Marek, M., Naiman-Sessions, M., Torres, J., & Morton, C. H. (2014). A report on the cross-National Survey of doulas. *Childbirth Educators and Labor and Delivery Nurses in the United States and Canada.* https://www.academia.edu/12969378/Maternity_Support_Survey_A_Report_on_the_Cross_National_Survey_of_Doulas_Childbirth_Educators_and_Labor_and_Delivery_Nurses_in_the_United_States_and_Canada

Shreffler, K. M., Tiemeyer, S., Dorius, C., Spierling, T., Greil, A. L., & McQuillan, J. (2016). Infertility and fertility intentions, desires, and outcomes among US women. *Demographic Research, 35*, 1149–1168.

Taouk, L. H., Fialkow, M. F., & Schulkin, J. A. (2018). Provision of reproductive healthcare to women with disabilities: A survey of obstetrician–gynecologists' training, practices, and perceived barriers. *Health Equity, 2*(1), 207–215.

Tsai, S., Shaia, K., Woodward, J. T., Sun, M. Y., & Muasher, S. J. (2020). Surrogacy laws in the United States: What obstetrician–gynecologists need to know. *Obstetrics & Gynecology, 135*(3), 717–722.

United Nations. (2019). *A human rights-based approach to mistreatment and violence against women in reproductive health services with a focus on childbirth and obstetric violence (advancement of women).* Issue. U. Nations. https://digitallibrary.un.org/record/3823698

Vedam, S., Stoll, K., Taiwo, T. K., Rubashkin, N., Cheyney, M., Strauss, N., McLemore, M., Cadena, M., Nethery, E., & Rushton, E. (2019). The giving voice to mothers study: Inequity and mistreatment during pregnancy and childbirth in the United States. *Reproductive Health, 16*(1), 1–18.

Villines, Z. (2019). The maternal mortality lie that ensures women will keep dying. *Daily KOS.* https://www.dailykos.com/stories/2019/10/23/1894584/-The-Maternal-Mortality-Lie-That-Ensures-Women-Will-Keep-Dying

Wingo, E., Ingraham, N., & Roberts, S. C. (2018). Reproductive health care priorities and barriers to effective care for LGBTQ people assigned female at birth: A qualitative study. *Women's Health Issues, 28*(4), 350–357.

Worthington, A. K., Burke, E. E., Shirazi, T. N., & Leahy, C. (2020). US Women's perceptions and acceptance of new reproductive health technologies. *Women's Health Reports, 1*(1), 402–412.

Chapter 5
Maternal Mental Health and Illness

Cheryl Tatano Beck

5.1 Current State of Maternal Mental Health Inequities in the USA

Disparities and inequities in severe maternal mortality and mortality exist with Black women compared to White women in the USA (Howell, et al., 2018; Petersen et al., 2019). These social and ethnic disparities persist despite researchers controlling for confounding variables, such as social and demographic factors related to adverse perinatal outcomes. Hoyert (2021) reported that maternal mortality rates for Black mothers are 3.5 times higher than White mothers and 2.5 times higher than Hispanic mothers. American Indian/Alaska Native mothers have almost as high a rate as Black mothers (United Health Foundation, 2021). Admon et al. (2021) investigated the trends in suicide 1 year before and after birth among insured childbearing women in the USA from 2006 to 2017. Black women, women with lower income, and younger women experienced larger increases in suicide over this time period.

Undiagnosed and untreated mental health of women related to childbirth is a silent health issue in the USA (Postpartum Support International, 2020). Reported rates of postpartum depression and posttraumatic stress bring much-needed attention to racial and ethnic disparities. For example, Liu and Tronick (2014) found that Black women in the USA had an up to two-fold greater rate of postpartum depression compared to White women. Lucero et al. (2012) reported that Hispanic women in the USA had a three times larger rate of postpartum depression than for the general American population. Women of color are more likely to experience postpartum depression compared to White women even after socioeconomic factors are

C. T. Beck (✉)
University of Connecticut, Storrs, CT, USA
e-mail: cheryl.beck@uconn.edu

© The Author(s), under exclusive license to Springer Nature Switzerland AG 2023
B. A. Anderson, L. R. Roberts (eds.), *Maternal Health and American Cultural Values*,
Global Maternal and Child Health, https://doi.org/10.1007/978-3-031-23969-4_5

controlled for (Liu et al., 2016). Blackmore and Chaudron (2014) identified prevalence rates for Hispanic women during the postpartum period that ranged between 12% and 59% for depressive symptoms and/or major depression. For women of Mexican descent, rates of postpartum depression may be as high as 50% (Lucero et al., 2012). In a review of 38 studies, the prevalence rate of postpartum depression in Asian women ranged from 8.2% to 70% (Koirala & Chuemchit, 2020).

Severe maternal morbidity involves experiences of life-threatening complications during childbirth and postpartum. Cardiovascular conditions such as cardiomyopathy and hypertensive conditions including pre-eclampsia and eclampsia are some main causes of severe maternal morbidity and death for Black women (Shahul et al., 2015). Maternal near miss is a term that refers to women who survive one of these life-threatening obstetric complications. Black women have twice the risk of experiencing a near miss compared to White women (Conrey et al., 2019; Leonard et al., 2019). Women with a maternal near miss reported experiencing postpartum depression as one of its long-term impacts (TorkmannejadSabzevari et al., 2021).

Even after controlling for confounding variables like sociodemographic factors, comorbidity, and obstetric factors, Black race placed women at a higher risk for severe maternal morbidity than White women (Howland et al., 2019; Leonard et al., 2019). There is a need for researching other explanations or pathways such as a focus on structural racism (Howland et al., 2019). Racism and not race needs to be considered as a key factor in helping to explain Black women's high risk for poor maternal health outcomes compared to White women (Canty, 2022). A misplaced assumption may be operating that it is race alone that places Black women at higher risk for severe maternal morbidity.

5.2 Social Determinants of Health: Social and Community Context

In *Healthy People* 2030, one of the domains under the social determinants of health (SDoH) is *social and community context* (Healthy People, 2030). Under this domain is *discrimination*, an unfair, socially structured action/stressor with a negative physiological effect.

Using data from the Pregnancy Risk Assessment Monitoring System (PRAMS), Segre et al. (2021) examined whether perceived racial discrimination was associated with postpartum depressed mood. In the sample (2013–2015; $N = 2805$), 4.4% of the women perceived racial discrimination with rates higher in Black and Hispanic perinatal women. Using logistic regression, this analysis revealed that perinatal women who had experienced perceived racial discrimination were twice as likely to report depressed mood compared to perinatal women who had not reported racial discrimination.

Weeks et al. (2022) also used data from the PRAMS and found that recent social discrimination was associated with almost three times higher odds of women of color experiencing postpartum depression symptoms. The prevalence of postpartum depressive symptoms in women of color was 14.7% compared to 10.4% among White women. Women of Color reported the prevalence of social discrimination was 12.2%. Black mothers had the highest prevalence of discrimination (18.1%), followed by Hispanic mothers (13.3%). Weeks et al. concluded that racism is a dangerous stressor for maternal mental health.

In a multisite study with 537 low-income Hispanic women in the USA, Ponting et al. (2020) reported that at one month postpartum, discrimination and domestic violence each were significantly related to higher postpartum depressive symptoms even when controlled for marital status, education, and negative life events.

Chan et al. (2021) examined racial and ethnic differences in rates of hospital-based care with respect to postpartum depression in California from 2008 to 2012. The primary outcome was *first postpartum hospital encounter with a diagnosis of depression* occurring within a 9-month period after birth. Rates of hospital-based care for postpartum depression were highest among Black women and lowest among Asian women compared to White women. Chan et al. suggest their findings identify an urgent need to investigate structural barriers and systemic issues related to mental healthcare that impact the higher rate of hospitalizations for Black women. Inpatient care should be the last resort for psychiatric care during the postpartum period.

Perceived healthcare bias and postpartum mental health during the COVID-19 pandemic were investigated with 237 women who gave birth in New York City. The sample consisted of 61.7% White women, 14.5% Hispanic, 12.3% Asian, 8.5% Black, and 3% other (Janevic et al., 2021). Women who were SARS-CoV-2 positive, Black, and Hispanic had higher perceived healthcare discrimination. Women who experienced healthcare discrimination had higher levels of postpartum stress and birth-related posttraumatic stress disorder (PTSD). When focusing on the reasons for differential treatment by race/ethnicity, 60% of Asian mothers, 38% of Black mothers, 25% of Hispanic women, and 2% of White women related their treatment to race/ethnicity.

Since Black women are three to four times more likely to experience life-threatening complications during childbirth leading to near misses (Petersen et al., 2019), they are at risk for experiencing childbirth as a traumatic event developing into posttraumatic stress. Markin and Coleman (2021) suggest that there is an intersection of racism and childbirth trauma with potential to impact maternal mental health.

Qualitative researchers are providing an insider's peak at racial and ethnic disparities in severe maternal morbidity (Canty, 2022; Wang et al., 2021). In Canty's (2022) phenomenological study of severe maternal morbidity among Black women, a prominent theme was that *race matters.* Women perceived their skin color played a role in the way they were treated in the healthcare system. Women viewed negative interactions with their maternity providers as a subtle form of racism. Some Black women shared that they experienced racial biases. Healthcare providers were at times dismissive of Black women's symptoms and this factor influenced the type of care they reviewed. Some women questioned if they received such limited information on their risk for severe maternal morbidity because clinicians assumed they did not care or could not understand.

Wang et al. (2021) conducted a qualitative study with women who experienced severe maternal morbidity. Focus groups were organized by self-identified race/ethnicity: Black, Latina, and Asian or White. Across all these focus groups, women described their childbirth experience as traumatic. As the rate of severe maternal morbidity is higher among women of color, this places them disproportionally at risk for developing PTSD. Bay and Sayiner (2021) reported in a sample of 550 women one month postpartum that the probability of experiencing postpartum depression increased four to five times among women with a high level of traumatic birth perception.

5.3 Personal Control: An American Cultural Value Affecting Maternal Mental Health

The key American cultural value that has the potential for long-term impact on maternal mental health is *personal control*. This cultural value for Americans focuses on a person's ability to control themselves and their environment. It includes a person's beliefs regarding the degree to which they can influence events in their lives. When it comes to one of the most important events in a woman's life, giving birth, her ability to control what happens during her labor and delivery is critical to her mental health. Feelings of loss of control while giving birth can impact the development of various postpartum mood and anxiety disorders, such as postpartum depression and PTSD due to traumatic childbirth.

In a grounded theory study of postpartum depression, Beck (1993) discovered that the basic social psychological problem women experienced was loss of control over their thought processes, emotions, and actions. There was not an aspect of their lives that they felt they had the ability to control. Women struggling with postpartum depression attempted to resolve the problem of loss of control by means of a four-stage process called *Teetering on the Edge*. This title referred to women walking a fine line every day between sanity and insanity when they were in the depths of depression. These stages consisted of (1) encountering terror, (2) dying of self, (3) struggling to survive, and (4) regaining control.

Despite mothers with postpartum depression desperately wanting to get out of their psychological pain, they had no control over it. As this woman shared, "I had no control and that was the really scary thing. I felt trapped. I felt like there was absolutely no way out of this hell. These horrible feelings weren't going to leave no matter how hard I tried" (Beck, 1992, p. 169). Loss of control also permeated mothers' interactions with their infants, illustrating the domino effect postpartum depression can have (Beck, 1996). Women described postpartum depression as physically overtaking their minds and bodies. Mothers wanted to reach out to their infants but as this quote depicts, they had no control. "I had no control over my own self-being, nothing, mind, soul, nothing. It basically controlled me. I wanted to reach out to my baby, yet I couldn't" (Beck, 1996, p. 100).

Uncontrolled anger was yet another aspect of their lives for which women had no control. Mothers used the metaphor of an erupting volcano to try to explain how their festering anger would at times erupt without their control, and they feared they could possibly hurt their infants and older children (Beck, 2020). The following quote captures this loss of control over their emotions and actions:

> At times, I felt like something was exploding in me. More than anything, it was anger. I would get really angry for no reason. There were times I was real thankful my husband was here to take care of the baby (Beck, 2020, p. 113).

In a metasynthesis of 18 qualitative studies on postpartum depression, Beck (2002) identified four overarching themes: (1) pervasive loss, (2) incongruity between expectations and the reality of motherhood, (3), spiraling downward, and (4) making gains. Pervasive loss of control permeated deep into the crevices of mothers suffering with postpartum depression. Loss of control of self, of relationships, and their *voice* were all aspects of loss of personal control in their lives.

Box 5.1 Four Perspectives Involved with Postpartum Depression

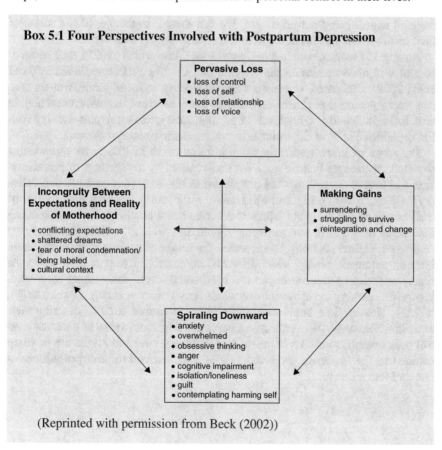

(Reprinted with permission from Beck (2002))

Postpartum onset of panic disorder is an anxiety disorder where loss of personal control is front and center (Beck, 1998). During panic attacks, mothers revealed that the terrifying physical and emotional components left them feeling totally out of control. As their panic attacks worsened, some mothers lost all sense of any control in their lives to the degree that some women had suicidal thoughts. This woman shared:

> I would write to my baby almost as if I knew I was going to die, which is morbid. I would write what I felt about him and how much I loved him. I think because in the back of my head I was always afraid. This is hard to say, but I think I was so out of control that I was afraid I might kill myself (quietly weeping) (Beck, 1998, p. 133).

One of the defining attributes of a traumatic birth is the terrifying loss of control (Beck, 2004a, 2015). Women who perceived their births as traumatic explained they lost all semblance of control over what was happening to them. Women shared that they felt their bodies were totally controlled by the labor and delivery staff. In active labor as women tried to cope with their increasingly strong contractions, they felt powerless and helpless to prevent what was being done to them. In a qualitative study, Meaney et al. (2016) found that women with severe maternal morbidity reported experiencing powerlessness. Women shared the uncontrollable nature of their severe complications of childbirth, unable to control their bodies.

Among 161 women who had cesarean births (Tomsis et al., 2021), their sense of control was measured using the Support and Control Birth questionnaire (Ford et al., 2009). Compared to women who had elective cesarean births, women who had emergency cesarean births experienced lower levels of internal control and, in turn, had significantly higher levels of posttraumatic stress symptoms. Loss of control explained 38.5% of the variance in posttraumatic stress symptoms.

For some mothers, traumatic childbirth can result in PTSD. As one woman depicted, "I strongly believe my PTSD was caused by my feelings of powerlessness and loss of control of what people did to my body [during labor and delivery]" (Beck, 2004a, p.33). In PTSD due to birth trauma, women lose control of their emotions and thoughts. Mothers describe being bombarded with distressing flashbacks of the birth and terrifying nightmares which they had absolutely no control over (Beck, 2004b). Women used the image of a video of their traumatic birth on automatic replay, which they had no control to stop or even pause. At times, women experienced anger at a heightened level. This mother recounted, "powerful seething anger would overwhelm me without warning" (Beck, 2004b, p. 221). Ticking time bomb was a phrase some women used to describe their uncontrollable anger. The strong and pervasive American value of personal control over oneself, one's environment, and influence over life events are in sharp contrast to the immense perceived loss of personal control and powerlessness among these mothers.

5.4 Summary

Disparities and inequities in maternal mortality and morbidity, specifically with regards to perinatal mood and anxiety disorders, exist with women of color compared to White women in the USA. In this chapter, the SDoH domain, social and community context, was chosen to explore why. Personal control, as a predominant American cultural value, plays heavily in the state of affairs of maternal mental health and illness. Postpartum depression has received the most attention by researchers, comparing the prevalence rates in women of color with White women. Only a couple of researchers are bringing attention to the intersection of racism and childbirth trauma. More research is definitely needed to tease out this connection. To date, no studies could be located that focused on any other perinatal mood and anxiety disorder in women of color, such as postpartum onset of panic disorder, postpartum obsessive-compulsive disorder, or postpartum psychosis.

Green et al. (2021) developed the cycle to respectful maternity care as an actionable framework to address maternal outcome disparities in Black women. The cycle to respectful care consists of seven phases: waking up, getting ready, reaching out, implementing with provider community, coalescing with local community, creating change, and maintaining. Data collected from focus groups and one-on-one interviews with Black women who had given birth in hospitals within the last 2 years were used to create this cycle. Core values of this cycle included:

- Value for Blackness.
- Birth equity.
- Reproductive justice.
- Professional oath.
- Holistic maternity care.
- Humanity.
- Love.

The cycle to respectful care is a reflection of the need to address the pervasive American cultural value of personal control. It can be applied especially to women of color during the childbearing process in a cultural environment where loss of personal control is highly stigmatized.

References

Admon, L. K., Dalton, V., Kolenic, G. E., Ettner, S. L., Tilea, A., Haffajee, R. L., Brownlee, R. M., Zochowski, M. K., Tabb, K. M., Muzik, M., & Zivin, K. (2021). Trends in suicidality 1 year before and after birth among commercially insured childbearing individuals in the United States, 2006-2017. *JAMA Psychiatry, 78*(2), 171–176. https://doi.org/10.1001/jamapsychiatry.2020.3550

Bay, F., & Sayiner, F. D. (2021). Perception of traumatic childbirth of women and its relationship with postpartum depression. *Women & Health, 61*(5), 479–489. https://doi.org/10.108 0/03630242.2021.1927287

Beck, C. T. (1992). The lived experience of postpartum depression: A phenomenological study. *Nursing Research, 41*(3), 166–171. https://doi.org/10.1097/00006199-199205000-00008

Beck, C. T. (1993). Teetering on the edge: A substantive theory of postpartum depression. *Nursing Research, 42*(1), 42–48. https://doi.org/10.1097/00006199-199301000-000082

Beck, C. T. (1996). Postpartum depressed mothers' experiences interacting with their children. *Nursing Research, 45*(2), 98–104. https://doi.org/10.1097/00006199-199603000-00008

Beck, C. T. (1998). Postpartum onset of panic disorder. *Image: Journal of Nursing Scholarship, 30*(2), 131–135. https://doi.org/10.1111/j.1547-5069.1998.tb01267.x

Beck, C. T. (2002). Postpartum depression: A meta-synthesis of qualitative research. *Qualitative Health Research, 12*, 453–472. https://doi.org/10.1177/104973202129120016

Beck, C. T. (2015). Middle range theory of traumatic childbirth: The ever-widening ripple effect. *Global Qualitative Nursing Research*, 1–13. https://doi.org/10.1177/2333393615575313

Beck, C. T. (2020). Mother-infant-interaction during postpartum depression: A metaphor analysis. *Canadian Journal of Nursing Research, 52*(2), 108–116. https://doi.org/10.117 7/2F0844562119897756

Beck. (2004a). Birth trauma: In the eye of the beholder. *Nursing Research, 53*(1), 28–35. https://doi.org/10.1097/00006199-200401000-00005

Beck. (2004b). Post-traumatic stress disorder due to childbirth: The aftermath. *Nursing Research, 53*(4), 216–224. https://doi.org/10.1097/00006199-200407000-00004

Blackmore, E. R., & Chaudron, L. (2014). Psychosocial and cultural considerations in detecting and treating depression in Latina perinatal women in the United States. In S. Lara-Cinisomo & K. Wisner (Eds.), *Perinatal depression among Spanish-speaking and Latin American women* (1st ed., pp. 83–96). Springer. https://doi.org/10.1007/978-1-4614-8045-7_6

Canty, L. (2022). The lived experience of severe maternal morbidity among black women. *Nursing Inquiry, 29*, e12466. https://doi.org/10.1111/nin.12466

Chan, A. L., Guo, N., Popat, R., Robakis, T., Blumenfeld, Y. Y., Main, E., Scott, K. A., & Butwick, A. J. (2021). Racial and ethnic disparities in hospital-based care associated with postpartum depression. *Journal of Racial and Ethnic Health Disparities, 8*(1), 220–229. https://doi.org/10.1007/s40615-020-00774-y

Conrey, E. J., Manning, S. E., Shellhaas, C., Somerville, N. J., Stone, S. L., Diop, H., Rankin, K., & Goodman, D. (2019). Severe maternal morbidity: A tale of 2 states using data from action-Ohio and Massachusetts. *Maternal and Child Health Journal, 23*(8), 989–995. https://doi.org/10.1007/s10995-019-02744-1

Ford, E., Ayers, S., & Wright, D. B. (2009). Measurement of maternal perceptions of support and control in birth (SCIB). *Journal of Women's Health, 18*, 245–252. https://doi.org/10.1089/jwh.2008.0882

Green, C. L., Perez, S. L., Walker, A., Estriplet, T., Ogunwole, S. M., Auguste, T. C., & Crear-Perry, J. A. (2021). The cycle to respectful care: A qualitative approach to the creation of an actionable framework to address maternal outcome disparities. *International Journal of Environmental Research and Public Health, 18*, 4933. https://doi.org/10.3390/ijerph18094933

Healthy People. (2030). U.S. Department of Health and Human Services, Office of Disease Prevention and Health Promotion. https://health.gov/healthypeople/objectives-and-data/social-determinants-health

Howell, E. A. (2018). Reducing disparities in severe maternal morbidity and mortality. *Clinical Obstetrics and Gynecology, 61*(2), 387–399. https://doi.org/10.1097/GRF.0000000000000349

Howland, R. E., Angley, M., Won, S. H., Wilcox, W., Searing, H., Liu, S. Y., & Johansson, E. W. (2019). Determinants of severe maternal morbidity and its racial/ethnic disparities in new York City, 2008-2012. *Maternal and Child Health Journal, 23*(3), 346–355. https://doi.org/10.1007/s10995-018-2682-z

Hoyert, D. L. (2021). Maternal mortality rates in the United States, 2019. Health e-stats. 2021 Issue. https://www.cdc.gov/nchs/data/hestat/maternal-mortality-2021/E-Stat-Maternal-Mortality-Rates-H.pdf

Janevic, T., Maru, S., Nowlin, S., McCarthy, K., Bergink, V., Stone, J., Dias, J., Wu, S., & Howell, E. A. (2021). Pandemic birthing: Childbirth satisfaction, perceived health care bias, and post-partum health during the COVID-19 pandemic. *Maternal and Child Health Journal, 25*(6), 860–869. https://doi.org/10.1007/s10995-021-03158-8

Koirala, P., & Chuemchit, M. (2020). Depression and domestic violence experiences among Asian women: A systematic review. *International Journal of Women's Health, 12*, 21–33. https://doi.org/10.2147/IJWH.S235864

Leonard, S. A., Main, E. K., Scott, K. A., Profit, J., & Carmichael, S. L. (2019). Racial and ethnic disparities in severe maternal morbidity prevalence and trends. *Annals of Epidemiology, 33*, 300–336. https://doi.org/10.1016/j.annepidem.2019.02.007

Liu, C. H., & Tronick, E. (2014). Prevalence and predictors of maternal postpartum depressed mood and anhedonia by race and ethnicity. *Epidemiology and Psychiatric Sciences, 23*(2), 201–209. https://doi.org/10.1017/S2045796013000413

Liu, C. H., Giallo, R., Doan, S. N., Seidman, L. J., & Tronick, E. (2016). Racial and ethnic dif-ferences in prenatal life stress and postpartum depression symptoms. *Archives of Psychiatric Nursing, 30*(1), 7–12. https://doi.org/10.1016/j.apnu.2015.11.002

Lucero, N. B., Beckstrand, R. L., Callister, L. C., & Sanchez Birkhead, A. C. (2012). Prevalence of postpartum depression among Hispanic immigrant women. *Journal of the American Academy of Nurse Practitioners, 24*(12), 726–734. https://doi.org/10.1111/j.1745-7599.2012.00744.x

Markin, & Coleman, M. N. (2021). Intersections of gendered racial trauma and childbirth trauma: Clinical interventions for black women. *Psychotherapy.* https://doi.org/10.1037/pst0000403

Meaney, S., Lutomski, J. E., O'Connor, L., O'Donoghue, K., & Greene, R. A. (2016). Women's experience of maternal morbidity: A qualitative analysis. *BMC Pregnancy and Childbirth, 16*, 184. https://doi.org/10.1186/s12884-016-0974-0

Petersen, E. E., Davis, N. L., Goodman, D., Cox, S., Syverson, C., Seed, K., Shapiro-Mendoza, C., Callaghan, W. M., & Barfield, W. (2019). Racial/ethnic disparities in pregnancy-related deaths - United States, 2007-2016. *Morbidity and Mortality Weekly Report, 68*(35), 762–765. https://doi.org/10.15585/mmwr.mm6835a3

Ponting, C., Chavira, D. A., Ramos, I., Christensen, W., Guardino, C., & Dunkel Schetter, C. (2020). Postpartum depressive symptoms in low-income Latinas: Cultural and contextual contributors. *Cultural Diversity & Ethnic Minority Psychology, 26*(4), 544–556. https://doi.org/10.1037/cdp0000325

Postpartum Support International. (2020). Mind the gap: A strategic roadmap to address America's silent health crisis: Untreated and unaddressed perinatal mental health disorders. *Mind the Gap National Report.* https://www.postpartum.net/mind-the-gap

Segre, L. S., Mehner, B. T., & Brock, R. L. (2021). Perceived racial discrimination and depressed mood in perinatal women: An extension of the domain specific stress. *Women's Health Issues, 31*(3), 254–262. https://doi.org/10.1016/j.whi.2020.12.008

Shahul, S., Tung, A., Minhaj, M., Nizamuddin, J., Wenger, J., Mahmood, E., Muellar, A., Shaefi, S., Scavone, B., Kociol, R. A., Talmor, D., & Rana, S. (2015). Racial disparities in comorbidi-ties, complications, and maternal and fetal outcomes in women with preeclampsia/eclampsia. *Hypertension in Pregnancy, 34*(4), 506–515. https://doi.org/10.3109/10641955.2015.1090581

Tomsis, Y., Perez, E., Sharabi, L., Shaked, M., & Haze, S. (2021). Postpartum post-traumatic stress symptoms following cesarean section-the mediating effect of sense of control. *Psychiatric Quarterly, 92*, 1839–1853. https://doi.org/10.1007/s11126-021-09949-0

TorkmannejadSabzevari, M., Yazdi, M. E., & Rad, M. (2021). Lived experiences of women with maternal near miss: Qualitative research. *The Journal of Maternal-Fetal and Neonatal Medicine, 35*, 7158. https://doi.org/10.1080/14767058.2021.1945576

United Health Foundation. (2021). *America's health rankings: Health of women and children.* United Health Foundation. https://www.americashealthrankings.org/explore/health-of-women-and-children/measure/overall_hwc_a/state/ALL

Wang, E., Glazer, K. B., Sofaer, S., Balbierz, A., & Howell, E. A. (2021). Racial and ethnic disparities in severe maternal morbidity: A qualitative study of women's experiences of peripartum care. *Women's Health Issues, 31*(1), 75–81. https://doi.org/10.1016/j.whi.2020.09.002

Weeks, F., Zapata, J., Rohan, A., & Green, T. (2022, Feb). Are experiences of racial discrimination associated with postpartum depressive symptoms? A multistate analysis of pregnancy risk assessment monitoring system data. *Journal of Women's Health, 31*(2), 158–166. https://doi.org/10.1089/jwh.2021.0426

Chapter 6
The Lived Experience of American Mothers in the Military

Lana J. Bernat

The views presented in this chapter are my own and do not necessarily represent the views of the Department of Defense or the United States Army.

LTC Lana J. Bernat, United States Army Nurse Corps

6.1 Mothers in the Military Culture

Mothers in the military community, while generally young and healthy, are under incredible stress as they navigate transient lifestyles, family separations, or single-parenting. They are often lonely, especially when family separations occur. Mothers have to navigate daily routines and special events such as birthdays and first days of school while either they or their partner is away for training or deployments. Working mothers in military communities may face challenges accessing quality childcare, and even greater challenges exist if they are on duty for 24-hour shifts or night shifts. Single parents or parents in dual military marriages experience additional strain from conflicting family and career demands. Mothers who deploy are exposed to additional stressors such as battlefield hazards and gender-related threats such as discrimination, harassment, and assault.

Mothers with deployed partners worry about their partner's health and safety. Studies show that military spouses of deployed Service Members have higher rates of mental health disorders such as depression, anxiety, and sleep disturbances, especially during periods of war (De Burgh et al., 2011). Often located far from their extended families, they must rely on other support systems to adapt to their unique challenges. In this chapter, I (LB) share my perspective on the lived experiences of

L. J. Bernat (✉)
U.S. Army Nurse Corps, Falls Church, VA, USA
e-mail: lana.j.bernat.mil@health.mil

© The Author(s), under exclusive license to Springer Nature Switzerland AG 2023   63
B. A. Anderson, L. R. Roberts (eds.), *Maternal Health and American Cultural Values*,
Global Maternal and Child Health, https://doi.org/10.1007/978-3-031-23969-4_6

American mothers in the military community. My perspective is informed through my personal experience as a military spouse and active-duty military mother as well as my professional care of military mothers as a nurse, case manager, and nurse-midwife. There are unique resources and hazards impacting the lived experience and the health outcomes of mothers in the military community. Self-reliance, a key American cultural value, is highly valued and provides a window into how these mothers cope with both the military culture and the military healthcare system.

Mothers in the military community are primarily categorized as military spouses or Service Members, referred to as uniformed mothers. In 2020, nearly 38% of the total military force had at least one child, so mothers account for a great portion of the military community. Many uniformed mothers are single parents or in dual-military marriages. As of 2020, approximately 19,000 uniformed mothers on active duty are single parents, and more than 22,000 uniformed mothers are in Guard and Reserve components. More than 32,000 active duty parents and more than 20,000 Reserve component members are in dual-military marriages (United States Department of Defense [DOD], 2021).

Mothers who serve on active duty or who are spouses of active-duty Service Members usually live on or near a military base. Active-duty families generally move every three years. With each move, the family has to start over with new schools, jobs, neighborhoods, and friends. Mothers who serve or who are military spouses to Service Members in Reserve units or Guard units generally live in civilian communities. Civilian communities lack the support and structure of military bases, and some Service Members travel a significant distance to attend monthly and annual training events. As a result, these mothers may experience even greater stress during periods of training or deployment because they are disconnected from support systems that exist on military installations (DOD, 2021).

6.2 Maternal Health Care in the Military Community

Military mothers have access to healthcare benefits through TRICARE, a uniformed services healthcare program. This program includes direct care through military hospitals, clinics and network care through civilian healthcare providers and institutions. There are two network care options: *Prime*, a managed care program equivalent to a civilian Health Maintenance Organization (HMO) and *Select*, a program equivalent to a Preferred Provider Organization (PPO) (Defense Health Agency, n.d., updated 10/13/2021).

While research on military mothers is limited and the military population is generally young and healthy, available data shows that some health outcomes are superior for mothers in the military community, compared with American mothers in general. The Military Health System (MHS) is among the leading health organizations in reporting low maternal mortality and morbidity. Between 2009 and 2018, pregnancy-related mortality in the MHS, including direct care and network care options, was 7.4 maternal deaths per 100,000 live births in comparison to the

National Perinatal Information Center (NPIC) rates of 11.3 maternal deaths per 100,000 live births (United States Office of the Secretary of Defense, 2019). Because the MHS is a universal healthcare model, it has been identified as a contributor to these excellent outcomes.

Koehlmoos and colleagues conducted a systemic review of 32 studies assessing racial disparities in healthcare within the MHS. They concluded that the universal health coverage within the MHS appears to mitigate many disparities in medical procedures and screenings (Koehlmoos et al., 2021). Some research questions this conclusion. A 12-month retrospective cohort study between 2018 and 2021 of more than 1000 births within the MHS showed significant disparities for Black mothers in regard to frequency of cesarean delivery, increased intensive care unit (ICU) admissions, and overall severe maternal morbidity (Hamilton et al., 2021).

Black mothers had a cesarean delivery rate of 31.68% compared to 23.58% for White mothers, although these are still low levels of cesarean birth compared to the general population of mothers in many areas of the United States (USA). The ICU admission rate among Black mothers (0.49% compared to 0.18% for White mothers) was almost three times higher and the incidence of severe maternal morbidity (2.66% vs. 1.66%) was higher, even without including blood transfusion, although there was no difference in overall postpartum hemorrhage. The researchers concluded that equitable healthcare access and socioeconomic status at time of delivery and within the milieu of the military community did not completely eradicate racial disparities. They proposed the social determinant of health (SDoH) of systemic racism as an area for further study (Hamilton et al., 2021).

6.3 The Evolving Family Culture in the Military

There are unanswered questions about the cultural influences, policies, and practices within the military communities? One such question is: what are the individual, family, and community SDoH that impact mothers in the military?

6.3.1 The Historical Expectations of Mothers in the Military Community

The family culture within the military has evolved over time. Historically, military policies have discouraged marriage, particularly for lower enlisted ranks. "If the Army wanted you to have a wife, they would have issued you one!" was a common adage in the early twentieth century, but World War II required a shift in thinking, as the government needed to provide family benefits to recruit and retain men (Covkin, n.d.). Concurrent with the American culture of that era, military wives were expected to be homemakers and mothers. There were limited other roles except for the nurses, mostly single, who provided nursing care for wounded or sick active duty Service Members. Military wives were viewed as an extension of their Service Member partner, expected to volunteer for social programs supporting military families. As in the general American culture, these role expectations have persisted in defining the lived experience of military mothers (Covkin, n.d.).

6.3.2   Contemporary Expectations of Mothers in the Military Community

Today, many partners of Service Members continue to volunteer for unit morale and family readiness activities. Volunteering may provide a sense of meaning and belonging. In some cases, these social connections lead to enduring friendships. However, they may volunteer because they feel pressured to do so for the benefit of their partner's career path. These pressures increase as their partners advance in their careers and frequently when active duty training or deployment occurs. I have personally witnessed the wives of senior ranking military impose great pressure on these partners, often mothers, to volunteer or engage in the military community. Through personal conversations I have learned that there is the *perception* among these partners of lower ranking Service Members that the spouse of a senior military can be influential in performance evaluation for career advancement, dependent upon their volunteer willingness. These pressures and concerns are part of the lived experience of mothers in the military community.

Until the 1970s, women were not allowed to serve in the military if they had children or became pregnant. There has been progress in improving career paths and policies for women in the military, including addressing the support of motherhood and parenting. Some examples are increasing parental leave to 12 weeks, offering training and deployment deferments, requiring quality lactation spaces in the workplace, and offering the option for continual military service with a career intermission while raising a family (Defense Health Agency, n.d.). Despite these substantial advances in policy, uniformed mothers still experience pressures that affect the decision and timing for procreation and lactation. Many uniformed mothers have told me that pregnancy still carries stigma in their military units. Examples of this stigma include rumors that she purposely got pregnant to avoid training or deployment rotations or coworkers expressing annoyance because childbearing causes duty limitations or work disruption for lactation breaks.

The military culture may also impact a uniformed mother's decision to seek care for issues unrelated to or subsequent to childbearing. For instance, some mothers have told me that urinary incontinence or pelvic pain has been dismissed. They have voiced concerns that seeking further care might restrict or potentially negatively impact career advancement. These perceptions of not being heard or potential threat to livelihood and career can discourage seeking care and adversely impact maternal health outcomes. Uniformed mothers who belong to Reserve or Guard units may face additional challenges when they deploy. While military communities are accustomed to deployment as a part of the job, civilian communities may not provide the support the mother needs. Culturally in the USA when a father deploys and leaves the children behind, it is often viewed as a heroic act for his country. Deployed mothers may face cultural backlash, media shaming, and stigma from the community, deeming them unfit and neglectful mothers.

6.3.3 Conflicts for Working Mothers in the Military Community

Working military spouse mothers, uniformed single mothers, or dual-military mothers experience significant challenges in balancing the demands from work and home. The DOD invests heavily in programs to support families. Ultimately, however, Service Members are responsible for ensuring the well-being of their family. When a family problem negatively impacts the Service Member's ability to work, then the unit leadership may get involved. Most military families want to avoid this intrusion by managing situations before it reaches the ears of commands and reflects negatively upon the Service Member. While this may foster self-reliance, it may place tremendous stress on the mother. It can contribute to under-utilization of available resources and increase potential for poor health outcomes.

Dual-military families experience unique stressors when both parents work. The mother in the military community, uniformed or not, is often viewed as the person primarily responsible for the home and the children. Some uniformed mothers have told me that when a father asks for time off to care of a sick child, his supervisor often asks why the mother cannot perform the task, even if she has equal or greater out-of-home work responsibilities. These kinds of situations contribute to stress and guilt especially among working mothers. Some have expressed that their lived experience includes an ongoing sense of inadequacy and failure in self-reliance at both home and work.

Dual-military mothers also face career planning challenges. For example, many uniformed mothers say that one member of the dual-military couple has to have priority, and their own career is often secondary to their partner's in order to ensure career advancement. This compromise may also be due to logistic limitations, if work at her level of competency is unavailable at the new assignment location. This problem is compounded by the frequency of moves, averaging every three years. The uniformed mother's career may also be impacted when there is a difficult family situation for which she is expected to take primary responsibility. If she then has prolonged or recurrent work absences, she may be deemed unworthy of career advancement.

The working mother whose partner is a Service Member also deals with career challenges because of the transient nature of military life, limited job opportunities in some locations, and the demanding hours of the Service Member. Despite military spouse employment programs, these mothers may have difficulty finding employment unless they accept entry-level positions. They may experience significant delays in finding childcare, contributing to unemployment and underemployment, impacting the family income stream. These mothers may feel isolated, with frequent shifts in location and loss of social connections. These challenges for mothers in the military community have been amplified by the COVID-19 pandemic.

6.3.4   Self-Reliance in the Military Community

Self-reliance, a strong American cultural value, enables mothers to survive and thrive even under harsh and stressful conditions. Self-reliance manifests as strong independence, confidence, and taking individual responsibility in seeking out information about resources and making decisions. It has long been an important cultural value in the military, as Service Members and their family members are expected to adapt under adversity and to care for themselves and their families. Conversely, self-reliance can become such a strong expectation that mothers who seek help, especially for mental healthcare, are stigmatized.

Military communities have many DOD-funded programs and services that aim to promote self-reliance. However, military policies have nether a formal definition nor a specific method for measuring self-reliance (Meadows et al., 2016) although a tool for assessing the self-reliance of military families in the absence of the Service Member was previously developed and validated (McCubbin et al., 1996). Acknowledging that self-reliance can be a barrier to mental healthcare, the RAND Center for Military Health Policy Research studied factors that promote psychological resilience. In this study, resilience was defined as successful adaptation in the context of risk and adversity. Researchers found strong evidence that positive thinking, coping, and affect positively impacted resilience. They also reported that family support and community connection contributed to resilience (Meredith et al., 2011).

6.4   The Military Community and the Social Determinants of Health

A unique SDoH facing mothers in the military community is the expectation that Service Members must be ready at all times for deployment, sometimes on short notice. Family readiness is an important component of military readiness, because the well-being of the family enables the Service Member to focus on the mission at hand. Self-reliance is key to family readiness, and this hinges on the mother's ability (uniformed or military partner) to tap into the resources—the programs and services that provide the support systems.

6.4.1   Promoting Family Readiness for Mothers in the Military Community

Resources for family readiness can be accessed through support centers on military bases or through a centralized website that supplements existing programs with a free, confidential, worldwide, 24-hour, 365 day/year access to a referral and information service (Military One Source, n.d.). Family readiness services are available for all military services as well as the National Guard and Reserve components. Services cross many domains, including career support, financial services, deployment support, and relocation or transition assistance. Services also include emergency family assistance, domestic abuse prevention and response, new parent support, nonmedical counseling services, and support for family members with special medical or educational needs. As life in the military community is demanding, it can create mental stress. The Morale, Welfare, and Recreational (MWR) program is included in family readiness (Military One Source, 2021a). The MWR program provides nearly 5000 different programs and services to promote health and foster community support systems (Military One Source, 2021b).

The military services have family readiness group structures that help disseminate information to military families and provide workshops that prepare volunteers to assist with family readiness functions. The communication pathways for family readiness groups are especially important when units are away for training or deployment. Units can use these channels to disseminate critical information, provide resources, and ensure there is a conduit for emergency situations (Military One Source, 2021a). In my experience, family readiness groups can create cohesion that helps families deal with separations and crises as exemplified in the following case study.

> **Box 6.1 Self-reliance does not mean being alone**
> As a military spouse, uniformed Service Member, and family readiness group leader, I have many recollections of mothers made stronger because of the bonds between military families. I will never forget the day that I sat in the chapel for a memorial service of a soldier killed in action. The couple was expecting a baby in just a few weeks, and we were there to support her. We military spouse mothers sat together, and it was a source of comfort during a difficult time as we not only felt concern for her, but also worried about our own spouses still engaged in combat. Near the end of the service, a gentleman walked through the chapel, playing Amazing Grace on the bagpipes and shortly after outdoor riflemen fired off rounds for the 21-gun salute. The music and the rifle shots took our breath away, and the entire row of women reached out to hold hands with one another. We were aware that the ache we felt in our chests was just a fraction of the loss she would feel forever. Those bonds stand the test of time, as many of us are still in touch decades later, including our beautiful sister. We have marveled at her strength in raising her daughter and continuing to honor the man who sacrificed his life for his country.
> (LTC Lana Bernat, DNP, CNM)

6.4.2 Promoting Self-Reliance for Mothers in the Military Community

Readiness programs and services seek to prevent adverse SDoH and promote self-reliance in the domains of economic stability, education, neighborhood, and community.

6.4.2.1 Economic Stability

Economic stability is promoted through steady paychecks, tax-free housing, subsistence stipends, and healthcare benefits. Mothers in the military community can experience mental health stress if there are unforeseen expenses, poor financial management, or problems with the paycheck distribution stream. However, food security as an SDoH is generally not an issue in comparison to the many low-income mothers in the general American population. As needed, military families, particularly those within the lower enlisted ranks, are eligible for federally-funded nutrition programs (Military One Source, 2021a).

6.4.2.2 Education

Education assistance programs for both uniformed mothers and military spouse mothers include tuition assistance, scholarships, and free career counseling services. Many military bases have libraries, and the MWR library program provides free access to a digital library, foreign language courses, genealogical databases, and an e-reference business and information technology library. There is a 24-hour, 7-day online tutoring program to support the education needs of military families (Military One Source, 2021a). These resources can foster self-reliance and build financial security for mothers in the military, especially those facing the separation of deployment of the Service Member. It can promote maternal mental health to be actively engaged in developing her own skills and talents as well as being a support to the Service Member.

6.4.2.3 Neighborhood and Community

The neighborhood and the built environment of military families differ by location and by the family's decision to live in on-base or off-base housing. Affordability, neighborhood quality and safety, and school ratings factor into a family's decision to live on- or off-base. Some families choose off-base living because they can purchase a home or have more options for rental homes. Families may also prefer more privacy, more integration with the local community, and enjoy some distance between work and home. Families living off-base have a housing allowance calculated upon level of pay grade and location. The amount of this allowance is periodically updated to keep pace with the local market. On the other hand, on-base housing offers immersion in the military culture, decreases financial burdens, provides more opportunities to connect with other military families, and offers convenient access to military base amenities. These amenities usually include grocery stores, small shopping centers, fitness centers, parks, swimming pools, bowling alleys, and other recreational activities. Overall, living on military bases is safer in comparison to other similarly-sized communities, mainly because these are gated communities with restricted access. Military base housing is managed through a privatized housing model, established by Congress, with the intent of improving the quality of life and improving housing conditions for military families (DOD, 2018; Military One Source, 2021a, 2021b). In recent years, however, I have witnessed that families have reported maintenance delays and problems with environmental hazards such as mold and lead.

High-quality affordable childcare is a crucial service for military families who are almost always stationed remotely from their extended families. Mothers in the military community, particularly uniformed mothers and working spouse mothers, need supportive childcare programs to balance employment and parenting demands. The availability of affordable, quality childcare affects the ability of uniformed mothers to continue serving in the military. Childcare centers with an income-based fee structure are generally located on the military base. Home-based child care options delivered by certified childcare military spouses may offer more flexible hours for working mothers. Hourly care and a limited amount of free monthly childcare hours may be available at some locations, but accessing this benefit may still be difficult. Placement for childcare is limited and many mothers have told me about long waiting lists and their concern about finding safe alternatives to on-base childcare centers. The military gives priority to single parents and dual-military parents (DOD, 2018; Military One Source, 2021a). However, even mothers who fall into these categories have shared their struggles with me about being able to arrange childcare before parental leave periods end.

Advances in technology and social media have expanded connections for military mothers. Most communities have formal and informal social media pages specific to their military base, where mothers share information and resources with one another and provide advice in problem-solving. In times of crisis, volunteers often emerge to help provide assistance, and I have seen this in action within social media communities. Seasoned mothers may offer respite childcare to a young, overwhelmed mother. When a mother posts about being new to the community, other mothers respond with offers to meet for play dates at the park or invitations to other social venues. A mother may post about the angry outbursts her spouse is exhibiting, and other mothers share experiences, resources, and support. Mothers in these online communities are bound by the common experience of a military lifestyle. Volunteer page administrators address violations of established ground rules for the group, which helps promote a safe psychological space for military mothers.

6.5 Summary

Mothers in the military community generally receive excellent healthcare and have lower maternal morbidity and mortality rates than the general population of American mothers. They do, however, endure high levels of mental stress from living transient lifestyles, dealing with family separations during training and deployments, or functioning in single-parent families in a military readiness environment. Stress, resulting from the social and community context, is an SDoH unique to the military. It is a significant pathway in which physical or social factors can contribute to poor maternal health outcomes. There is, however, a safety net in the military community with robust resources. The military community embraces the American cultural value of self-reliance. While the military community encourages mothers in the military community to engage in self-reliance, this cultural values can also be a barrier for accessing care. Mothers in the military who struggle with self-reliance, especially with psychiatric needs and accessing mental health services, may experience stigmatization, contributing to less than optimal maternal health outcomes.

References

Covkin, S. (n.d.). *A short history of U.S. Army wives, 1776-1983*. U.S. History Scene. Open access. https://ushistoryscene.com/article/a-short-history-of-u-s-army-wives-1776-1983/

De Burgh, H., White, C., Fear, N., & Iversen, A. (2011). The impact of deployment to Iraq or Afghanistan on partners and wives of military personnel. *International Review of Psychiatry, 23*, 192–200. https://doi.org/10.3109/09540261.2011.560144

Defense Health Agency. (n.d.) *Tricare health plans,* updated 10/13/2021. https://www.tricare.mil/Plans/HealthPlans

Hamilton, J., Shumbusho, D., Cooper, D., Fletcher, T., Aden, J., Weir, L., & Keyser, E. (2021). Race matters: Maternal morbidity in the military health system. *American Journal of Obstetrics, 224*, 512e1–512e6. https://doi.org/10.1016/j.ajog.2021.02.036

Koehlmoos, T., Korona-Bailey, J., Janvrin, M., & Madsen, C. (2021). *Racial disparities in the military health : A framework synthesis*. Military Medicine. https://doi.org/10.1093/milmed/usab506

McCubbin, H., Thompson, A., & McCubbin, M. (1996). *Family assessment: Resiliency, coping and adaptation: Inventories for research and practice*. University of Wisconsin.

Meadows, S., Beckett, M., Bowling, K., Golinelli, D., Fisher, M., Martin, L., Meredith, L., & Osilla, K. (2016). Family resilience in the military: Definitions, models, and policies. *RAND Health Quarterly, 5*(3), 12. https://www.rand.org/pubs/periodicals/health-quarterly/issues/v5/n3/12.html

Meredith, L., Sherbourne, C., Gaillot, S., Hansell, L., Ritschard, H., Parker, A., & Wrenn, G. (2011). Promoting psychological resilience in the U.S. military. *RAND Health Quarterly, 1*(2), 2. https://www.rand.org/content/dam/rand/pubs/monographs/2011/RAND_MG996.pdf

Military One Source. (2021a). *Military family readiness system*. https://www.militaryonesource.mil/family-relationships/family-life/keeping-your-family-strong/military-family-readiness-system/

Military One Source. (2021b). *About morale, welfare, and recreation: Supporting the military community.*   https://www.militaryonesource.mil/military-life-cycle/friends-extended-family/about-mwr-morale-welfare-and-recreation/

Military One Source. (n.d.). *About us.* https://www.militaryonesource.mil/about-us/

United States Department of Defense. (2018, Dec 13). Charter. Military Family Readiness Council. https://download.militaryonesource.mil/12038/MOS/MFRC/MFRC-Charter-2018-2020.pdf

Part III
Mothers in a Divided Nation

Chapter 7
Immigrants, Refugees, and Undocumented Mothers

Barbara A. Anderson and Lisa R. Roberts

7.1 Privilege of Place

Home, including family, community, and nation, is the place of belonging, privilege, safety, and personal control. Personal control is a culturally transmitted belief about the degree to which one can shape one's life, positively or negatively. Disruptions in place of belonging can occur for many reasons. Intimate partner violence is a common cause of disruption and loss of personal control within the immediate environment (Anderson et al., 2002). Community level violence, natural and man-made disasters, political persecution, genocide, and war can disrupt place of belonging and devastate any sense of personal control (Anderson & Anderson, 2020). These events can result in internal displacement within a nation, such as Hurricane Katrina, or it can result in migration beyond national borders. However, this is not necessarily related to untoward events.

Migration is movement to another nation of which one is not a citizen in order to achieve a specific goal, often with the intention of settlement as a permanent resident or naturalized citizen. It may occur in efforts to improve economic standards, to form family relationships across nations, to pursue career opportunities, or for safety. All persons seeking settlement within another country are *immigrants*. *Refugees* are a category of immigrants defined by the United Nations High Commission for Refugees (UNHCR) as "…people who have fled war, violence or persecution and have crossed an international border to find safety in another country" (UNHCR, n.d., para 1). These persons are eligible, upon the discretion and invitation of other nations, to settle in and seek citizenship in these nations. Examples

B. A. Anderson (✉)
Frontier Nursing University, Versailles, KY, USA

L. R. Roberts
Loma Linda University, Loma Linda, CA, USA

© The Author(s), under exclusive license to Springer Nature Switzerland AG 2023
B. A. Anderson, L. R. Roberts (eds.), *Maternal Health and American Cultural Values*,
Global Maternal and Child Health, https://doi.org/10.1007/978-3-031-23969-4_7

are recent invitations by the USA to selected Afghan and Ukrainian refugees. Most immigrants have legal documentation of entrance into the USA. Immigrants who entered without legal immigration papers or continued residence beyond a specified time frame without renewing legal immigration papers are defined as *undocumented immigrants* (Department of Homeland Security, n.d.). As of 2018, 86.4 million people in the USA, about 27% of the population, were immigrants or their children, who were often citizens by birth in the country (Zong et al., 2018, Feb 8). Immigrants may or may not be warmly welcomed.

7.2 Motherhood and Place

Many immigrants face difficulties in accessing healthcare and navigating both cultural differences and legal requirements in the healthcare system (Lawrence et al., 2020). Having a sense of personal control is influenced by place and being an immigrant in an unfamiliar environment can be daunting. Difficulty accessing adequate maternal healthcare can increase their risk for poor maternal health outcomes (Aptekman et al., 2014; Banke-Thomas et al., 2017; Hasstedt et al., 2018; Kentoffio et al., 2016; United States Preventive Services Task Force, 2021).

An immigrant mother's sense of personal control is influenced by her lived experiences, cultural norms from both her country of origin and the USA, and perceived self-efficacy in controlling one's self and environment. Whether legal, refugee, or undocumented, she may feel may feel overwhelmed, at least temporarily, in a new country. Having left any or all of her former social, economic, cultural, and linguistic ties may create disruption to sense of place (Ogbuagu, 2021; Pangas et al., 2019). Perceived personal control and sense of place as the first hurdles in seeking care can potentially delay entrance to care (Jain et al., 2022).

Utilizing care includes gaining entry to a healthcare site and developing a patient–provider relationship (Gulliford et al., 2002; Millman, 1993). Finding a provider who can meet her physical needs, but who engenders trust and is culturally humble and respectful may not be so easy (Banke-Thomas et al., 2019). English or Spanish proficiency may or may not be an issue. Some immigrants have not had an opportunity to access such linguistic education in their home countries (Banke-Thomas et al., 2017; Deacon & Sullivan, 2009). Lack of insurance and/or economic or social resources are also considerable hurdles (Banke-Thomas et al., 2019; Deacon & Sullivan, 2009; Hacker et al., 2015; Hasstedt et al., 2018). Complex paperwork, bureaucracy, institutional policies about coverage, limited safety net services, discriminatory practices, negative provider and staff attitudes, high-intervention models of birthing, media charges of extortion, and fear of deportation and/or interruption of the immigration process can affect sense of personal control and impede access to care (Banke-Thomas et al., 2019; Cabral & Cuevas, 2020; Hacker et al., 2015; Hasstedt et al., 2018; Heckert, 2020; Jain et al., 2022; Ogbuagu,

2021; Pangas et al., 2019). Many fear being labeled as a "public charge" if they apply for public assistance (Lawrence et al., 2020). Many immigrant mothers fear and do experience disrespectful care or abusive treatment (Pangas et al., 2019; United Nations, 2019, July 11).

Upon entrance to the USA, some immigrants have superior health indicators. This is termed the *immigrant paradox*. These excellent health indicators erode the longer the immigrants are in the USA. Some explanations for this are described as follows. First, there is a general expectation that all immigrants are in dire straits, certainly not the case. There may be selection bias in that healthier immigrants have the energy to go to another nation. The "salmon bias" is the description of sicker immigrants who return to their natal countries. Lastly, is the well-researched finding of dietary, social and family changes within one generation of immigration, often resulting in increased consumption of low-nutrient fast foods and alcohol use as well as decreased family involvement and support (Lawrence et al., 2020).

The immigrant paradox may or may not affect birth outcomes. The immigrant paradox seems to hold for Mexican-immigrant mothers who have better birth outcomes in the first generation. Conversely, birth outcomes among South Indian mothers are worsened by immigration. Immigrant mothers are very diverse, from those entering the USA in good health and with legal immigration status to those who are suffering from acute and chronic conditions, malnutrition, and the stigma of refugee or undocumented status (Lawrence et al., 2020). Overall, immigrant women are at increased risk for specific pregnancy and birth-related complications including postpartum depression, gestational diabetes, induction, and cesarean delivery (Hasstedt et al., 2018; Shellman et al., 2014). Nonetheless, mothers who immigrate to the USA often do so voluntarily (Volkan, 2018), indicating a propensity for adaptation and personal control. Programs such as the Oregon's expansion of Emergency Medicaid to cover undocumented immigrant women have shown a positive effect on maternal health outcomes as these mothers have been encouraged to exercise personal control in their healthcare (Swartz et al., 2019). While all immigrants face numerous unknowns in a new country, each faces challenges in adapting to the healthcare system.

7.3 Exemplars of the Lived Experience

We, BA and LR, have both worked for many years providing healthcare to immigrant, refugee, and undocumented mothers in the USA and in international settings. We offer a few composite exemplars of personal control among the many resilient and courageous women with whom we have worked.

7.3.1 Exemplar: An Immigrant Mother from South Asia

Mothers from South Asian countries may face limited autonomy in healthcare decision-making. In traditionally patriarchal societies, men often decide if and when a family member should be taken to a healthcare facility and what decisions should be made about care. After immigrating to the USA, these mothers may experience some confusion as healthcare providers ask them to make at least minor decisions at the point of care, and may be unprepared to do so without consulting family members. As a nurse practitioner, I (LR) have encountered mothers from South Asia with little autonomy and personal control who embraced personal control as empowering. Ruma, a 23-year-old mother from Bangladesh, was pregnant with her fourth child when I met her. She was distraught due to the difficult birth of her third child and stated she had barely recovered when she became pregnant again. She expressed fear regarding her impending delivery and caring for her other children, expecting during another prolonged recovery and even another pregnancy. Our rapport developed over several visits and as the time drew closer to her due date, Ruma and I discussed options for future birth control. She listened carefully and accepted the printed information I provided, saying she would try to discuss the matter with her husband. Ruma had never initiated any conversation pertaining to family planning with her husband. To consider doing so now was both exhilarating and intimidating, but a first step toward personal control in adapting to her new environment.

7.3.2 Exemplar: An Immigrant Mother from the Middle East

Mothers from the Middle East may demonstrate personal control by requesting a female provider and maintaining both physical and cultural modesty at all times. However, as a social expectation often demanded by male partners, this may not always be a matter of personal control for the mother. Salma came to me (LR) at three weeks postpartum with significant weight loss following the birth of her first child, a beautiful baby girl. Her husband expressed concern and frustration. He said "She does not eat, then she is weak and cannot care for our child properly." Initially, he was reluctant to leave the room, stating he would interpret for her, although Salma spoke English. The baby was fussy and he left the room with her. Salma then tearfully explained that she did not feel she was a good mother. She had anticipated being overjoyed with motherhood, but instead said she felt miserable with little interest in doing anything. Salma screened positive for postpartum depression. She was referred for care, but her husband insisted upon a female provider and refused the referral when they learned that a female psychologists or psychiatrist was not immediately available. Salma would not broach the subject of referral with her husband and continued to be depressed and unresponsive to her child, husband, and environment. The necessity of a female psychologist, psychiatrist or psychiatric nurse practitioner in this situation was essential.

7.3.3   Exemplar: A Refugee Mother from Southeast Asia

Refugees face unique challenges in seeking and accessing healthcare (Banke-Thomas et al., 2019) and in feeling safe in their new environment. The dictates of the culture, however, may provide significant strengths. I (BA) spent five years doing ethnographic research with Cambodian refugees in the refugee camps and border camps in Thailand and the third country resettlement areas of Southern California. I conducted doctoral and postdoctoral research on the health-seeking behaviors and practices of Cambodian refugee mothers. Like other southeast Asian populations, the role of women in the family is strong. Women are the designated healthcare guardians for family members including infants, children, adolescents, their male partners, the elderly who need assistance, and themselves. They have autonomy in their care. The women, especially the senior females, have a strong voice in determining who is considered sick (or not), what traditional treatments should be prescribed, and whether allopathic medicine is acceptable. These women have significant control over what happens. They have definite opinions on how to manage the 40-day lying-in period after childbirth including the treatment of *mother roasting* (charcoal burners or space heaters under the bed to warm the body even in 100 F degree heat in Southern California), the avoidance of any dietary *cold* foods (ice water, fruits and vegetables), and the importance of *hot* foods (meat, meat broths, and rice wine). After her baby was born, Radina was very upset when the nurse encouraged her to drink the ice water provided at her bedside, telling me the nurse was trying to murder her. The strengths in the culture gave her voice to express her concern and the personal control to explain why this was so upsetting (Anderson & Frye, 1989; Anderson & Frye, 1995).

7.3.4   Exemplar: A Second-Generation Mother from Central America

I (BA) checked my list of patients at the Southern California inner-city clinic not far from the Mexican–US border where I was a nurse-midwife provider. Thirty patients on the list, a wide diversity of both English- and Spanish-speaking mothers. Many were long-established as citizens, others were immigrants in process of obtaining citizenship or green cards, and some were undocumented. California had made the decision to offer maternity care to all women regardless of immigration status. This clinic was not far from the canyon described in the book *The Tortilla Curtain* (Boyle, 1996), a thinly-veiled novel that riveted the nation with narratives of devastating outcomes for undocumented persons, including pregnant women.

On the list, Rosa was identified as a 16-year-old primigravida, a confirmed first pregnancy. When I went into the exam room to meet Rosa, another woman in her mid-30 s sat beside her, nursing a toddler. Rosa introduced me to her mother, Navidad, and her little brother, Enrique. Navidad was a first-generation immigrant, originally entering the country with undocumented status, and eventually becoming a citizen. Rosa was a citizen, having been born in the USA, along with seven of her nine siblings. She had just completed her sophomore year in high school when she became pregnant. The baby's father was a high-school dropout who worked as a mechanic but economics were tight. Gang membership offered financial opportunities and community status. Francisco, nicknamed Paco, sometimes came with Rosa to her prenatal visits and was very proud of becoming a father. Rosa planned to breastfeed her baby, as her mother had with all her children, and she was honored within the family for her healthy pregnancy. She wore her maternity clothes as tightly as possible to shown off the developing curvature of her pregnancy.

I cared for Rosa during childbirth, a short and gentle labor with minimal intervention and the birth of a well-developed baby boy ready for his first meal. While Rosa labored during the wee hours of the night, Paco was caught in the crossfire of gang violence and killed in a shoot-out on the mean streets of the night. Rosa was devastated but held her little son close to her bosom, nursing him with the skills she has learned from her own mother. She assumed control of her life, enfolded within the safe arms of family-her *madre, padre, tios, tias, sobrinos,* and all the rest of the extended family.

7.4   Undocumented: The Shadow World of the 70-Mile Rio Grande Valley

The Rio Grande River of southern Texas and the vast deserts of the southwest are legendary in American history. The border between Mexico and the USA, stretching across Texas to California, is a place that is a culture unto itself. There are pockets of violence, as described in the graphic novel *No Country for Old Men* (Cormac McCarthy, 2006). Undocumented immigrants usually enter the USA at one of these points. The Rio Grande Valley (RGV) has a fluctuating population as it is a frequent wintering site for agricultural migrant workers who fan across the vast agricultural lands in the USA during planting and harvesting times.

Annually, migrant field workers from Mexico and Central America come to the rural Midwestern farmlands and to the Central Valley of California in the USA to harvest the crops. Their arrival to pick tomatoes was part of my rural Midwestern childhood. As a child, I (BA) played with their children in the migrant camps, fascinated by the sound of their melodic Spanish as we traded English and Spanish words. There were many pregnant women in the migrant camps. They worked in the fields even as labor started. When one mother went into labor, I ran home to tell my mother. By the time we arrived, the baby was born. My mother took the young woman and her baby to the local doctor who proclaimed both to be in good health. It was not until far ahead in the future that I learned the harsh realities that faced these migrant mothers.

Later, as a university professor, I learned about a project located in the Rio Grande Valley (RGV) in southern Texas near the US–Mexico border. They offered maternity care for all mothers, legally documented or otherwise. Holy Family Services, founded in 1983 by four Roman Catholic nuns, is a licensed free-standing birth center operated by Certified Nurse Midwives (CNMs). It has been licensed longer than any other birth center in Texas (see https://www.holyfamilybirthcenter. com/about-us). Some of my students went there for clinical rotation and one of my former doctoral students, Dr. Heather Swanson, became the director. While in Texas, I asked her if I could visit Holy Family in the Rio Grande Valley. She invited me to stay on site and learn about the holistic approach to maternity care that included full-scope care as well as lodging and food for birthing families as needed, gardening projects promoting home gardening, assistance with immigration paper-work, and opportunities for volunteers. Holy Family definitely understands that adverse social determinants of health (SDoH) can drive maternal health outcomes and structures to program to help families have healthy outcomes in an environment of respectful maternity care.

In this chapter, we (BA & LR) examined personal control as an American value that affects mothers on the southern border. We interviewed Dr. Ann Millard, PhD, professor of anthropology and public health in the RGV and former editor of the *Medical Anthropology Quarterly* and Dr. Heather Swanson, DNP, CNM, professor of nursing and former director of Holy Family Services. They both generously shared the rich tapestry of their experiences in this unique American landscape.

7.4.1 The Path to Personal Control

The sense of personal control may be eroded by immigration, especially if under the intense stress of crossing the border undocumented. Many undocumented immi-grants have walked across the Rio Grande river, but at times it becomes turbulent and deep, resulting in drowning deaths. Others have crossed through the deserts of the Southwest. Undocumented immigrants may take high risks as they flee incred-ibly dangerous situations. That characterization does not apply to all immigrants, but a common thread among immigrants is seeking options, choices, and control in their lives.

Dr. Ann Millard (AM) observed that the undocumented women initially seem to lose their sense of autonomy in their lives. She described young mothers, sheltered initially by Catholic Charities USA Center on the border, as being very subdued and fearful of what would happen next as they witnessed local retaliation against the center. In providing sanctuary, Catholic Charities USA has experienced a significant number of hate messages and personal threats directed toward the Catholic Sisters (Clarke, 2022, Feb 16). As immigrants establish a new life initiating the documenta-tion processes, spreading out into the community to create a living environment, and coming together as communities (*colonias*), they begin to grow in a sense of per-sonal control. She described this process of establishing a new life as fraught with difficulty—finding a place to live, obtaining the necessities for survival, and reestablishing traditional spheres of influence and responsibility. They struggle with significant SDoH: economic instability with transient employment, language barriers, lack of health literacy, lack of adequate family support and sometimes violent neighborhood conditions. They fear calling the police as they negotiate the legal documentation process. Dr. Millard stated, "It's enough to drive anybody crazy, the amount of pressure to be in a society when you don't have documents and it's just gotten worse over the years" (AM, personal communication, August 9, 2022).

She also described a thoughtful process in which careful resource management and acceptance of less-than-ideal living conditions is accepted as a path to personal control. Often, a family rents or informally buys a piece of unimproved land lacking sewage, water, trash removal, and electricity. Family composition fluctuates as those in agricultural migrant work come in and out. They accept low-paying transient jobs as a path to increased job security and personal control. Mothers may be left behind to manage the properties while others seek agricultural work. Gradually they improve the property although any financial setback can destroy all gains. In general, nutrition erodes with time, tending toward junk food. Most families do not plant a home garden for food security as gardening is perceived as a marker of poverty (AM, personal communication, August 9, 2022).

Pregnancy and childbirth at the Southern Border is influenced by the mother's legal status, border politics, a healthcare system at times besieged by danger in the streets, and the deeply rooted culture of honoring motherhood. Dr. Heather Swanson (HS) described maternity care in the RGV. Some families choose to obtain maternity care at low-cost unlicensed clinics providing birth services. The licensed healthcare workforce is comprised primarily of physicians, many of whom are Hispanic-Americans as well as a significant number from the Indian subcontinent who have immigrated to the USA, certified nurse-midwives, and professional nurses, many of Hispanic-American heritage. It is essential for these healthcare providers to be fluent in Spanish. Maternity care is offered in clinics and hospitals and there is high-turnover among healthcare providers due to burnout and the large volume of care provided. Some mothers have private or public insurances but for undocumented persons, much of the financial transactions are cash or barter. Families in the process of negotiating legal status must provide ongoing financial records to case workers and they fear disclosure of any unpaid bills that could impede the movement toward legal status. Holy Family Services is a licensed freestanding birth center offering full-scope maternity care for nonsurgical deliveries provided by nurse-midwives. Families are offered additional services such as assistance with the necessary immigration paperwork, the option of a safe environment and food for families on site during childbirth, and cash payment and sometimes barter (HS, personal communication, August 10, 2022).

There are many reasons for undocumented mothers and their families to be fearful. There is mistrust and the sense that the healthcare system is cold and detached, yet they generally will not confront nor question medical decisions. Instead, they may ignore directions or spread the word about specific untrustworthy healthcare providers. Fearing ridicule, they may not be forthcoming about the *botanicas* and other traditional remedies that are commonly used nor will they discuss *susto,* a culture-bound syndrome describing fear and withdrawal behavior when one cannot cope (AM, personal communication, August 9, 2022; HS personal communication, August 10, 2022). In working with a comparable population in California, I (BA) found I needed to be very careful to ask about traditional practices and beliefs in a nuanced and nonjudgmental manner.

Providing and obtaining care during birth can be problematic for both healthcare providers and their clients. While data is somewhat limited, the cesarean rate is very high, up to 60% in some hospitals and fluctuating according to local conditions. In some areas, healthcare providers fear violence and abduction by violent gangs if they come into or leave the hospitals in some areas during hours of darkness. Clients in labor at night fear going into the streets to get to the hospitals. They will make huge efforts to reach a hospital early in the day to avoid street violence. Some doctors will do a quick cesarean section before leaving the hospital at sunset in order to get the baby born, similar to the dynamics in Bagdad, Iraq, during the height of the war there. Hospitals usually do not allow family, especially children, to stay with the laboring mother, particularly during the COVID-19 pandemic. Feeling "like a number in the system," restrained by finances or lack of emergency government Medicaid funding, isolated in labor, and concerned about safety after dark, many mothers and their families embrace the Holy Family model of care. If they are not a good fit for a low-risk birth in a free-standing birth center or they experience a complication during labor requiring transfer to a hospital, they frequently object. A typical comment in this situation is: "No, No, No—I can't pay the bill. I need to stay here because my immigration process is almost done and I can't show I owe any money and where will my family go?" In an emergency situation, and if no night ambulance is available or affordable (a frequent occurrence), a staff from the Holy Family may need to accompany the mother to the hospital. (HS, August 10, 2022). Enhancing the mother's sense of personal control is critical to helping her to embrace her role, to prevent psychological birth trauma, and avoid posttraumatic stress disorder, a common occurrence among mothers in the RGV (Heckert, 2020; Pangas et al., 2019; Shellman et al., 2014; Trainor et al., 2020; Volkan, 2018).

7.4.2   The Pathway to Inclusion

Personal control involves feeling included. The pathway to inclusion in the American culture may be strewn with experiences of exclusion, development of skills necessary for participation, overcoming adverse SDoH, and finding a balance between cultures. The experience of inclusion in the 70-mile checkpoint zone of the RGV may be quite different from other parts of the nation. Many undocumented and fully documented immigrants state that life in the 70-mile checkpoint zone buffers the social exclusion sometimes experienced in other parts of the nation (HS, personal communication, August 10, 2022). In the RGV, the Mexican-American culture is normative. There are robust indicators of cultural influence from the Mexican open-markets and small grocery stores, music, food trucks serving traditional cuisine, and large outdoor family gatherings with closely spaced children. Young women proudly display their pregnant bellies with tight and colorful clothing. It is customary to have photographs taken in late pregnancy to memorialize a serene, Madonna-like young mother with her enlarged pregnant abdomen (AM, personal communication, August 9, 2022; HS, personal communication, August 10, 2022). In California, I (BA) have been included in baptisms as an adult guardian (*comadre*), weddings, and celebration of *quinceañera*, the rite of passage acknowledging a young woman's coming of age at age 15. In the RGV and in much of the Southwest, these are normative events that promote a sense of inclusion and celebrate motherhood, but this inclusion is not necessarily experienced in all parts of the nation. As Dr. Swanson notes, "In most places along the 70 mile range, it is not really Texas or America. It's a different world that is a cultural merging" (HS, personal communication, August 10, 2022).

Feeling included and a sense of personal control in the 70-mile range is different from feeling inclusion in the larger American society. It may take significant time, especially for those who begin their journey in more difficult circumstances. One pathway to inclusion is education, highly respected among the Latinx immigrants of the RGV and elsewhere in the nation, even as they struggle with English language fluency and accessing educational opportunities for their children. Skills are valued and young men are encouraged to complete high school and then learn a skill, often manual, that will provide economic security, thus ameliorating the adverse SDoH, economic insecurity. Young women, often childbearing at a young age and with children in tow, are encouraged to complete high school and then pursue a tangible skill, such as bookkeeping or medical assistant. If a young woman becomes a medical assistant, donning the scrubs she wears to the clinic, the family expresses pride (AM, personal communication, August 9, 2022; HS, personal communication, August 10, 2022).

The Deferred Action for Childhood Arrivals (DACA) is a program initiated under the Obama Administration in 2012 to protect undocumented immigrants brought to the USA as children under the age of 16. Called the Dreamers Act, DACA has sought to provide a pathway for educational support and inclusion in American society for around 800,000 undocumented children as they emerged into adulthood (see https://www.uscis.gov/DACA). There have been many legal challenges to DACA, deepening political divisions in the nation.

Two powerful dramas are exemplars of the struggles of Latinx youth as they approach adulthood and parenting in America. The 2002 film, *Real Women have Curves*, captures the intergenerational conflict between an 18-year-old woman who wants to go to college and her traditional mother who wants her to marry and start childbearing. It is particularly poignant in depicting the issues of social inclusion and role expectations for young immigrant women. The 1988 documentary *Stand and Deliver* speaks to the issues around DACA, highlighting the struggles for sense of inclusion among undocumented immigrants. Based upon the true story of Jaime Escalante, a math teacher at an inner city high school in Los Angeles, it tracks his preparation of poorly prepared students from families in poverty to success in the national Advanced Placement Calculus exam. This story is exemplar of the pathway to inclusion facing undocumented immigrants—a pathway strewn with exclusion, development of skills necessary for participation, overcoming adverse SDoH, and finding the balance between cultures. Later, I (BA) was privileged to have taught two of Jaime Escalante's former students at the university graduate level. It was clear that these young Latinx students had overcome formidable SDoH and incorporated a sense of personal control. Likewise, undocumented immigrant mothers face challenges to personal control on their pathway to inclusion and healthy motherhood.

7.5 Summary

Having a sense of personal control is influenced by place. Being in an unfamiliar environment can be daunting and immigrant, refugee, or undocumented mothers may struggle with a sense of personal control in their journey toward inclusion in American society.

Many immigrants demonstrate the immigrant paradox, arriving in the USA with better health habits than second and subsequent generations. Adverse SDoH such as difficulty accessing adequate healthcare, health literacy, and a sense of safety and inclusion within the community all factor into the immigrant struggle, increasing the risk for poor maternal health outcomes. The challenge is to support those immigrants who become part of our society to maintain healthy behaviors and minimize risks for poor maternal health outcomes.

References

Anderson, E. N., & Anderson, B. (2020). *Complying with genocide: The wolf you feed*. Rowman & Littlefield Publishing Group.

Anderson, B. (Frye, B.) (1989). Health care decision making among Khmer immigrants Unpublished doctoral dissertation, Loma Linda University School of Public Health.

Anderson, B., & Frye, B. (1995). Use of cultural themes in promoting health among southeast Asian refugees. *American Journal of Health Promotion, 9*, 4.

Anderson, B., Hopp Marshak, H., & Hebbeler, D. (2002). Identifying intimate partner violence at entry to prenatal care: Clustering routine clinical information. *Journal of Midwifery and Women's Health, 47*, 5.

Aptekman, M., Rashid, M., Wright, V., & Dunn, S. (2014). Unmet contraceptive needs among refugees: Rossroads clinic experience. *Canadian Family Physician, 60*(12), e613–e619.

Banke-Thomas, A., Gieszl, S., Nizigiyimana, J., & Johnson-Agbakwu, C. (2017). Experiences of refugee women in accessing and utilizing a refugee-focused prenatal clinic in the United States: A mixed methods study. *Global Women's Health, 1*(1), 14–20.

Banke-Thomas, A., Agbemenu, K., & Johnson-Agbakwu, C. (2019). Factors associated with access to maternal and reproductive health care among Somali refugee women resettled in Ohio, United States: A cross-sectional survey. *Journal of Immigrant and Minority Health, 21*(5), 946–953.

Boyle, T. (1996). *The tortilla curtain*. Penguin Random House.

Cabral, J., & Cuevas, A. G. (2020). Health inequities among latinos/hispanics: Documentation status as a determinant of health. *Journal of Racial and Ethnic Health Disparities, 7*(5), 874–879.

Clarke, K. (2022). Two nuns have a message for Catholics angry about their ministry to immigrants: 'We don't have any intention of stopping. *America: The Jesuit Review*. https://www.america-magazine.org/politics-society/2022/02/16/catholic-charities-catholic-vote-migrants-242408

Cormac McCarthy, C. (2006). *No country for old men*. Vintage International.

Deacon, Z., & Sullivan, C. (2009). Responding to the complex and gendered needs of refugee women. *Affilia, 24*(3), 272–284.

Gulliford, M., Figueroa-Munoz, J., Morgan, M., Hughes, D., Gibson, B., Beech, R., & Hudson, M. (2002). What does' access to health care'mean? *Journal of Health Services Research & Policy, 7*(3), 186–188.

Hacker, K., Anies, M., Folb, B. L., & Zallman, L. (2015). Barriers to health care for undocumented immigrants: A literature review. *Risk Management and Healthcare Policy, 8*, 175.

Hasstedt, K., Desai, S., & Ansari-Thomas, Z. (2018). Immigrant women's access to sexual and reproductive health coverage and care in the United States. *Issue Brief (Commonwealth Fund), 2018*, 1–10.

Heckert, C. (2020). The bureaucratic violence of the health care system for pregnant immigrants on the United States-Mexico border. *Human Organization, 79*(1), 33–42. https://doi.org/10.17730/0018-7259.79.1.33

Jain, T., LaHote, J., Samari, G., & Garbers, S. (2022). Publicly-funded services providing sexual, reproductive, and maternal healthcare to immigrant women in the United States: A systematic review. *Journal of Immigrant and Minority Health, 24*(3), 759–778. https://doi.org/10.1007/s10903-021-01289-2

Kentoffio, K., Berkowitz, S. A., Atlas, S. J., Oo, S. A., & Percac-Lima, S. (2016). Use of maternal health services: Comparing refugee, immigrant and US-born populations. *Maternal and Child Health Journal, 20*(12), 2494–2501.

Lawrence, D., Ramakrishnan, K., & Yun, K. (2020). Achieving health equity for immigrants and their children. In A. Plough (Ed.), *Culture of health in practice: Innovations in research, community engagement, and action* (pp. 137–153). Oxford University Press.

Millman, M. (Ed.). (1993). *Access to health care in America*. National Academies Press. https://pubmed.ncbi.nlm.nih.gov/25144064/

Ogbuagu, B. C. (2021). Reimagining the convoluted plights of refugee, immigrant and undocumented immigrant women: Implications for the reauthorizations of the violence against Women's act of 1994 in the United States. *Social Education Research*, 75–102.

Pangas, J., Ogunsiji, O., Elmir, R., Raman, S., Liamputtong, P., Burns, E., Dahlen, H. G., & Schmied, V. (2019). Refugee women's experiences negotiating motherhood and maternity care in a new country: A meta-ethnographic review. *International Journal of Nursing Studies, 90*, 31–45.

Shellman, L., Beckstrand, R. L., Callister, L. C., Luthy, K. E., & Freeborn, D. (2014). Postpartum depression in immigrant Hispanic women: A comparative community sample. *Journal of the American Association of Nurse Practitioners, 26*(9), 488–497.

Swartz, J., Hainmueller, J., Lawrence, D., & Rodriguez, M. (2019). Oregon's expansion of prenatal care improved utilization among immigrant women. *Maternal and Child Health Journal, 23*(2), 173–182.

Trainor, L., Frickberg-Middleton, E., McLemore, M., & Franck, L. (2020). Mexican-born women's experiences of perinatal care in the United States. *Journal of Patient Experience, 7*(6), 941–945. https://doi.org/10.1177/2374373520966818

United High Commission for Refugees. (n.d.). *What is a refugee?* https://www.unhcr.org/en-us/what-is-a-refugee.html

United Nations. (2019). *A human rights-based approach to mistreatment and violence against women in reproductive health services with a focus on childbirth and obstetric violence,* United

Nations General Assembly 74th session: Advancement of women. https://digitallibrary.un.org/record/3823698

United States Department of Homeland Security. (n.d.). Reporting Terminology and Definitions. https://www.dhs.gov/data

United States Preventive Services Task Force. (2021). *A & B Recommendations*. https://www.uspreventiveservicestaskforce.org/uspstf/recommendation-topics/uspstf-a-and-b-recommendations

Volkan, V. D. (2018). *Immigrants and refugees: Trauma, perennial mourning, prejudice, and border psychology*. Routledge.

Zong, J., Batalova, J., & Hallock, J. (2018). Frequently requested statistics on immigrants and immigration in the United States. *Migration Information Source Spotlight*. www.migrationpolicy.org/article/frequently-requested-statistics-immigrants-and-immigration-united-states

Chapter 8
Maternal Health Outcomes and Othering: The Impact of Ethnicity and Race

Rachel S. Simmons

8.1 Historical Impact of Othering

The intersectionality of race, class, socioeconomic status, and culture has shaped Black motherhood perceptions (Owens, 2017; Harper, 2021; Rosenbaum, 2022; & Simmons, 2021). These phenomena have been based upon devastating myths and racism derisorily applied to Black women. Since 1619, when Africans tortuously arrived in America, Black motherhood has been associated with challenges. Black mothers were separated from their children and kinship bonds through the malignant and systemic structure of slavery. Throughout the eighteenth and nineteenth centuries, slavery genres and myths abounded (Hannah-Jones, 2021). Black women were stereotyped as having bio-psycho-socially incompatible human traits, thus lacking the virtues innately interrelated with maternal instincts. Black women were not granted the full dignity of autonomous motherhood as their culture was stripped from them and they experienced violations around conception, childrearing and breastfeeding. Mothers, forced into hard labor, also became commodities to support the corrupt system of slavery through production of babies. Unable to control their own destinies, Black mothers' identities were fragmented and disjointed, and many became ambivalent about motherhood—as the child was not their own (Greco, 2016). Currently, the American social construct of motherhood influencing public opinion on fitness for motherhood and role designation marginalizes many Black mothers into the category of *other*.

Black mothers are heterogeneous and experience *othering* in various ways across their lifespan. Adolescents, mothers in poverty, and single mothers are particularly disenfranchised by society through inequitable social determinants (health, employment, education) structurally incompatible with their needs as mothers. While Black

R. S. Simmons (✉)
Southwest Orlando Family Medicine, Orlando, FL, USA

© The Author(s), under exclusive license to Springer Nature Switzerland AG 2023
B. A. Anderson, L. R. Roberts (eds.), *Maternal Health and American Cultural Values*,
Global Maternal and Child Health, https://doi.org/10.1007/978-3-031-23969-4_8

women face different challenges related to motherhood, most share the lived experience surrounding the effects of slavery. This experience is shadowed by racism, prejudice, coercive social power, misapplied legislative authority, segregation, discrimination, and marginalization. History haunts the *othered* and hampers them in the quest for autonomous motherhood. Inequities, which still exist, stem from erroneous race-based science and medicine during the era of slavery. The preservation of oral tradition and storytelling in the Black community is a defense mechanism giving Black mothers control through astute discernment and hypervigilance regarding healthcare inequalities (Owens, 2017).

Black mothers have been susceptible to the will of *status quo* groups, loss of personal control, and unique barriers in accessing healthcare. Vast disparities exist in healthcare delivery, breastfeeding support, and managing the social determinants of health (SDoH). While the American cultural value around motherhood promotes personal control, it is often elusive for mothers who are *othered*.

8.2 Loss of Personal Control: The Lived Experience of Black Mothers

The American cultural value of personal control asserts that individuals can choose to have control over themselves, their environment, and their destinies. Individuals are assumed to have personal power to make informed choices for good or poor health. This assumption is not historically aligned with Blackness, pungently conflicting with the lived experiences of many Black mothers who continue to live with the historical effects of slavery. Adverse SDoH are not always amenable to personal control. Value conflict about personal autonomy creates cognitive dissonance and ambivalence about motherhood among Black mothers.

8.2.1 Ambivalence About Conception

Deciding *when* to have a child has historically been out of the control of Black women. During slavery, Black women often conceived and birthed children outside of their control, primarily due to de facto sexual violence. Because of extremely unequal power dynamics, there were minimal reproductive rights for Black women. The decision to *conceive* and *mother a child* was often entwined with the slave owners' financial needs, as many infants were commercialized. It was not uncommon for Black mothers to give birth and have the child taken away immediately or shortly after birth and sold into a life of slavery. The systemic process of "conception to slavery" left many Black mothers in anguish, leading to ambivalence about conception and motherhood. Ambivalence became a defense against the inevitability of loss of control and loss of the child (Greco, 2016).

Data from the Centers for Disease Control and Prevention (CDC) National Vital Statistics System indicated that while provisional birth rates for 2021 increased by 2% among non-Hispanic White and Hispanic women, the birth rate for non-Hispanic Black mothers declined by 2% (Hamilton et al., 2022, May). Yet, a cohort study of women *not desiring* children at the time of intercourse found that Black women were less likely to use contraception than other groups. Economic level and access to healthcare were not implicated as factors. Social mobility and locus of reproductive control were identified as variables needing further research (Grady et al., 2015). Motherhood ambivalence may be a plausible explanation for women who are *othered.*

Locus of reproductive control is a variable for *all* women in retaining or regaining autonomy over conception. The right to prevent unwanted pregnancy has been challenged and, if these challenges are successful, will likely disproportionately impact the *othered,* placing these women at further risk for undesired pregnancies and poor maternal outcomes (Finer & Zolina, 2016; Webb, 2022).

8.2.2 Ambivalence About Abortion

Abortion, as a central tenant of personal choice, was recently curtailed in the U.S. Supreme Court when *Roe v. Wade*, as a constitutional right, was overturned on June 24, 2022 (Roe v. Wade, 1973). This ruling will disproportionately impact the *othered* by further diminishing personal control and autonomous decision-making. *Othered* women's bodies remain the purview of reproductive injustice that White patriarchal legislative systems have long controlled. Recent infographics indicate that *othered* women are more likely to live in states with restrictive choice for abortion and limited support programs for mothers, children, and families (Rosenbaum, 2022). Further, Black mothers, especially those impacted by poverty, are highly impacted due to limited access and timeliness of care (Rosenbaum, 2022; Webb, 2022).

8.2.3 Ambivalence About Childrearing

Black women have been stereotyped as inadequate mothers by historical racist tropes originating during slavery and consistently reinforced from segregation to Civil Rights up to contemporary feminist eras. The infamous mammy caricature assigned to Black mothers dually acknowledged their childrearing and nurturing capabilities while disavowing their fitness for mothering. Negative imagery and appellations by politicians and even prominent Black leaders portrayed Black mothers as *careless breeders*, not accounting for sexual violence and extreme poverty (Harper, 2021).

Out of necessity for survival, many employed Black mothers accepted the role of matriarchal family head of household but then were subsequently labeled as "unfit mothers" for balancing both employment and motherhood. The absence of Black males in the home, stemming from structural policies that discriminated against male employment and upheld inequitable justice systems, reinforced the proverbial stereotype of the Black woman as "head of the household." Black mothers who were not working outside of the home or without adequate financial means to fully provide for their children were labeled "unfit for childrearing." Legislative policies developed to target these mothers included random drug testing, government assistance programs that excluded male residence in the home, and proposed sterilizations (Harper, 2021). The Black mother, as *othered*, was reduced to being a recipient of a monthly government stipend. The constant trolling about lack of fitness for motherhood leads to ambivalence about childrearing. Despite these messages and the ambivalence surrounding motherhood, Black mothers have shown incredible resilience.

8.3   Breastfeeding Exploitation Among Black Mothers: Historical and Contemporary Effects

Othered women were often denied autonomous decision-making about breastfeeding. The physical and psychological dignities surrounding breastfeeding were not granted to Black mothers and their infants. While breastfeeding, they were often harassed, sexually exploited, or forced to put multiple infants to their breasts at once. Furthermore, enslaved Black mothers' breastmilk was a commodity controlled and managed by relevant stakeholders. Black mother's milk provided nourishment and life for immeasurable numbers of Black and White infants. Historically, countless Black women reported breastfeeding most of their lives (Franklin & Moss, 2000).

Enslaved Black mothers were responsible for arduous field and housework while also having breastfeeding responsibilities. When breastmilk was required for White infants because their mothers were unable or unwilling to breastfeed, enslaved mothers, also known as wet nurses, were responsible for providing milk to sustain the infant's life. *Wet nursing* is the practice of breastfeeding an infant or infants other than one's biological child, a practice all over the world, generally in situations of duress. Wet nursing of multiple infants frequently led to diminished milk production or lactation failure. When milk production decreased or lactation failure occurred, the White infant was prioritized and wet nursing by lactating members of the enslaved community was the only means of saving the Black infant (Franklin & Moss, 2000). Enslaved Black slave mothers who failed to lactate sufficiently as ordered for a White infant were often beaten or sold away from kinship bonds.

Wet nursing, as part of enslavement, is scarcely mentioned in the literature. However, some works give credence to the trauma of enslaved wet nursing. Thus, there has been a prolonged cultural aversion to breastfeeding among the American Black population, grounded in the psychologically traumatic past when breastfeeding was commodified through violence and loss of autonomy (Berlin et al., 1996; Johnson et al., 2015; Jones-Rogers, 2017; Simmons, 2021).

Intergenerational trauma theory supports the concept that trauma may be genetically passed from one generation to the next through delayed gene expression, prenatal exposure, and repetitive injury from cultural, psychological, and socioeconomics dynamics (Fairfax, 2020; Yehuda & Lehrner, 2018). Black mothers continue to initiate and sustain breastfeeding at the lowest rate among American mothers. Black mothers initiate breastfeeding at 73.9% compared to 81.9% for White mothers. At six months, approximately 47.8% of Black mothers are still breastfeeding versus 60.6% of White mothers (Meier et al., 2010). The unprecedented baby formula shortage of 2022 impacted Black mothers disproportionately and highlighted the critical need to support efforts to breastfeed (Schreiber, 2022, May 24). Addressing cultural and systemic bias and promoting autonomous decision-making are essential.

The effects of trauma can be studied through participant observation, semistructured interviews, artifact review, and proximity to the informant group. Simmons (2021) conducted a qualitative ethnographic study exploring the culture of breastfeeding education at geographically diverse Historically Black Colleges and Universities (HBCU) on the mainland and outside mainland USA. A portion of the study focused on diverse Black nurse educators teaching Black undergraduate nursing students about breastfeeding. The findings identified that Black nurse educators, who possessed appropriate theoretical and clinical knowledge to teach undergraduate students about breastfeeding, were socio-culturally concordant with the lived breastfeeding experiences of *othered* mothers.

Despite having adequate knowledge of breastfeeding and a clear understanding of the benefits, some American Black nurse educators focused on the cultural challenges of breastfeeding due to racism, employment, and inadequate family support. By contrast, nursing educators outside the USA mainland supported breastfeeding as an innate mothering right, a finding also identified in global slavery research. Nursing educators living on the USA mainland from the northern and southern areas of the country cited ambivalence, broken culture, insecurity, racism in the healthcare system, and fear of breastfeeding in public due to unwanted sexual advances. These were also the challenges that faced enslaved mothers. This study suggests that intergenerational trauma described and experienced by Black nurse educators stems from chronic breastfeeding exploitation of *othered* mothers (Simmons, 2021).

Breastfeeding trauma appears to reside below the psyche of *othered* women—regardless of economic level. The author (RS) has witnessed and validated this trauma phenomenon across the life span while caring for *othered* women. This trauma appears to manifest through ambivalence or aversion to breastfeeding that prevents *othered* women from reaching personal lactation goals and following national guidelines. In order to assist Black mothers in breastfeeding, the author recommends fully integrating the SDoH in breastfeeding education including cultural awareness and systemic barriers (Simmons, 2021).

8.4   *Othered* Women and the Social Determinants of Health

The *Healthy People 2030* document describes the SDoH and focuses on five over-arching domains needed to decrease health risks and improve quality-of-life out-comes. The SDoH represent an individual's environment which impacts health outcomes and overall quality of life (Healthy People, 2030). *Othered* women face challenges beyond their personal control while residing in a system of norms, roles, and cognition that were designed, implemented, authenticated, and validated within a White environment (Feagin, 2006). Chronic systemic racism with inequitable structures that contribute to disparity often makes interventions for adverse SDoH very difficult.

8.4.1   *SDoH Domain: Health Care Access and Quality*

Healthcare, particularly in terms of quality and equity, has been deficient for most *othered* women. Racism originating from fallible science, practices, theories, and speculation during slavery still pervades healthcare (Owens, 2017). *Othered* moth-ers have been subjected to unethical and inhumane experiments as medical doctors desired to learn more about the female reproductive system with White women as the benefactors (Owens, 2017). Various obstetric and gynecological procedures and surgeries were performed on enslaved women without consent or anesthesia. Many enslaved women died from heart attacks, stroke, hemorrhage, or infection as a result (Owens, 2017).

Historically, the health and value of enslaved Black women was often deter-mined by medical doctors who assisted slave traders in making "informed" pur-chases and "investments" based on invalid hypotheses. Black women were medically determined to have higher pain thresholds having survived torturous beatings, hav-ing thicker skin as *evidenced* by keloids forming over traumatized skin, and the physical strength akin to men in performing arduous field labor (Owens, 2017). The need for survival was not considered during the assessment of the psychophysiolog-ical composition of the *othered*. Historical narratives from *othered* women support endurance and will to survive (Franklin & Moss, 2000). For many *othered* mothers, the maintenance of kinship bonds made the insufferable to some extent tolerable, particularly with their children in mind.

Distorted medical knowledge remains pervasive in our healthcare system and gravely impacts the quality of care that Black mothers receive. Correct knowledge and understanding are required to reduce maternal morbidity and mortality. Federal and state governments have worked to some extent to ensure access to healthcare, but the quality of care has long been debated and challenged by *othered* women. Black women have consistently complained about poor quality of care, as evidenced by not receiving adequate therapeutic effects from medications, being the subject of rude commentary, and not being actively heard. Disparity researchers have objectively validated persistent concerns regarding the quality of healthcare for *othered* persons (Hoffman et al., 2016; Owens, 2017; Simmons, 2021).

Studies show that Black women are the least likely to receive pain medicine relative to their White counterparts (Anderson et al., 2009; Anderson & Roberts, 2019; Meghani et al., 2012; Todd et al., 2000). Physicians' pain perceptions and treatment for Black persons with pain have shown to be disparate (Staton et al., 2007). This perception and lack of treatment indicate implicit bias and overcorrection in treating the pain of White persons (Hoffman et al., 2016). It is an internalization (conscious or unconscious) of nineteenth-century erroneous science. Though medical students are exposed to learning about implicit bias and medical injustice, studies indicate a persistent correlation between a strong belief in significant biological differences between Blacks and Whites and medical perceptions of diminished levels of pain among Blacks (Anderson & Roberts, 2019; Hoffman et al., 2016). A majority of students also believe that Blacks have thicker skin than Whites, thus less sensitive nerve endings (Staton et al., 2007; Hoffman et al., 2016).

Most healthcare providers seek to provide evidence-based care for the *othered*, but the quality of care may be dubious. The *othered* not only *desire* to *be cared for* but also yearn to *feel cared for* in healthcare. The profession of nursing, while highly trusted by the public, has demonstrated examples of pervasive racism, perhaps more dangerous than physician racism because of the time spent with and proximity to the patient (American Nurses Association [ANA], 2022). The juxtaposition of false beliefs and poor quality of care create a context for healthcare injustice with disparities, higher health costs, increased morbidity and mortality, and mistrust of the system (Healthy People, 2030; Owens, 2017).

8.4.2   SDoH Domain: Neighborhood and Built Environment

Neighborhoods and built environments have a major impact on the health and well-being of individuals (CDC, 2018). The lingering effects of redlining, a discriminatory practice of disinvestment in the neighborhoods of certain races and ethnicities, continue to segregate communities across the nation. Since investments are less likely to be made in these communities, low-income minorities reside in hollowed neighborhoods with inadequate housing, food, drinking water, poor air quality, and limited access to clinics and hospitals. *Othered* mothers are more likely to live in health and food deserts that impact overall health and well-being. For instance, the recent mass shooting in Buffalo, New York, highlighted a food desert community, as the massacre took place at the only full-service retailer in the area. Additionally, many *othered* mothers in rural communities suffer adverse birth outcomes and poor maternal health outcomes due to living in maternity care deserts (Purser et al., 2022). Neighborhoods and the built environment also impact maternal susceptibility to maternal complications from diabetes, hypertension, and heart disease (Anderson & Roberts, 2019).

8.5   The Impact of *Othering* on Maternal Health Outcomes

The duality of being Black and female presents disparate and unequal health impacts for the *othered*. Structural and individual racism, marginalization, and discrimination increase allostatic load, making chronic conditions disproportionately increased for the *othered*.

8.5.1   Allostatic Load

Allostatic load refers to the daily stressors that accumulate over time resulting in negative health manifestations. Homeostasis is repeatedly disrupted as the body attempts to self-regulate and repair. Among the *othered*, persistent stressors manifest as low morale, fatigue, exhaustion, and breakdown, due to constant erosion resulting from racism, marginalization, and discrimination. Thus susceptible, othered person's body will become ill or worn out by repeated injury. Increased rates of mental illness, hypertension, coronary artery disease, stroke, and diabetes are disproportionate in the *othered* and theorized to transpire from persistent allostatic loading.

Decades of statistics in the USA show Black women having poor maternal health outcomes. In 2020, the Centers for Disease Control and Prevention (CDC) reported the maternal mortality rate as 55.3 deaths per 100,000 live births for Black mothers. This rate is almost three times that of non-Hispanic and Hispanic mothers although American Indian and Alaska Native (AI/NA) mothers are not far behind (Hoyert, 2022). The devastating maternal health outcomes for Black mothers is complex and multifactorial, stemming from quality, access, timeliness of care, and provider-patient racial concordance.

The effects of structural racism and allostatic load outside of the purview of personal control have finally been accepted as a major contributor to poorer health among *othered* women including Black mothers (ANA, 2022; Anderson & Roberts, 2019; CDC, 2018; Hoffman et al., 2016; Owens, 2017; Staton et al., 2007; Webb, 2022).

8.5.2   Invisibility

Upon learning of being pregnant, many Black mothers, even those who have given birth before, fear navigating prenatal and birth care. They worry about lack of personal control or fear of disrespect from healthcare providers. They also worry about potential morbidity and mortality risks facing them.

Many *othered* mothers report feeling invisible when receiving healthcare: "African Americans are treated differently," "different women have different options," "every time I went to an appointment, it felt that I was being treated like a medical condition," and "it should not matter what type of insurance you have, everyone should be treated the same way with the same care" (Patruno, 2015, November 26). These heartbreaking narratives represent the lived experiences of many *othered* mothers who have experienced micro and major daily aggressions contributing to their allostatic load. Black mothers, seeking to mitigate the effects of discrimination, have begun to narrate their childbearing experiences and to share their birth stories. These stories may include feeling ignored when in severe pain or giving birthing without an attending healthcare provider because of staff shortages or lack of timely attention.

8.6   Racial and Cultural Concordance in Black Mothers

Racial and cultural concordant healthcare, provided by a person of parallel race and culture, suggests improved health outcomes and satisfaction for many Black mothers. The *othered* seek providers who will validate their lived experiences and provide culturally-based care. In fact, the proximity of racial and cultural concordance may be a matter of life or death for the *othered*. Greenwood et al. (2020) explored the concept of physician-patient racial concordance and the impact on clinical outcomes. An analysis of almost two million births in Florida from 1992 to 2015 identified that Black newborns treated by White physicians experienced 430 more fatalities per 100,000 births as compared to those treated Black physicians. This devastating finding suggests that cultural concordance may reduce health disparities and mortality in extreme circumstances (Greenwood et al. 2020). Regardless of clinical outcomes, Black mothers may have lower satisfaction with care and experience poorer communication in racial and cultural discordant contexts (Shen et al., 2018).

White mothers may also struggle with discordance with the race and culture of their healthcare providers, as they may have difficulty equating "Black" with doctor or healthcare provider. A recent study indicated that the perception of White patients to their response to healthcare treatments is influenced by the race and gender of their provider. This randomized controlled study showed that White patients were less physiologically responsive to the exact treatments administered by Black providers as compared to Asian and White providers. The notion of a Black provider is distant in the psyche of many White individuals, as evident by the reduced perception of physiological responses (Howe et al., 2020).

High social economic status is not a protective factor against bias for Black female healthcare providers who may be perceived as being *others*. Black female doctors are not always accepted by Whites though patients generally described feeling cared for by these providers (Anderson & Roberts, 2019; Howe et al., 2020). As the number of Black healthcare providers and culturally humble clinicians of all races seek to understand implicit bias and practice culturally-based care, the paradigm will begin to shift.

8.7 Summary

Othering among American childbearing women, particularly Black mothers, is nuanced. *Othered* mothers have significant lived experiences outside of society's norms; therefore, assimilation is not an option. Historical and contemporary systemic racism, discrimination, marginalization, and fragmented care make *othering* dangerous and even lethal for Black mothers. While they possess generational perseverance and resilience, they still lack full power to combat the systemic discrimination that impacts maternal health outcomes. The American value of personal control is elusive for many *othered* mothers whose health and well-being are pawns in an inequitable system.

References

American Nurses Association. (2022). *New survey data: Racism within the nursing profession is a substantial problem.* https://nursingworld.org/news-releases/2021/new-survey-data-racism-in-nursing

Anderson, B., & Roberts, L. (2019). *The maternal health crisis in America: Nursing implications for advocacy and practice.* Springer.

Anderson, K., Green, C., & Payne, R. (2009). Racial and ethnic disparities in pain: Causes and consequences of unequal care. *Journal of Pain, 10*(12), 1187–1204.

Berlin, L., Favreau, M., Miller, S., & Kelley, R. (1996). *Remembering slavery: African Americans talk about their personal experiences of slavery and emancipation.* The New Press.

Centers for Disease Control and Prevention. (2018). *Social determinants of health: Know what affects health.* https://www.cdc.gov/socialdeterminants/index.htm

Fairfax, C. (2020). The need to be since 1619, trauma and anti-blackness. *Phylon, 57*(1), 56–75. https://doi.org/10.2307/26924987

Feagin, J. R. (2006). *A theory of oppression.* Routledge.

Finer, L., & Zolina, M. (2016). Declines in unintended pregnancy in the United States. *New England Journal of Medicine, 374*, 843–852. https://doi.org/10.1056/NEJMsa1506575

Franklin, J., & Moss, A. (2000). *From slavery to freedom: A history of African Americans* (8th ed.).

Grady, C. D., Dehlendorf, C., Cohen, E. D., Schwarz, E. B., & Borrero, S. (2015). Racial and ethnic differences in contraceptive use among women who desire no future children, 2006-2010 National Survey of family growth. *Contraception, 92*(1), 62–70. https://doi.org/10.1016/j.contraception.2015.03.017

Greco, G. (2016). *Othering the mother: Traumatic effects of motherhood on the formulation of identity in Toni Morrison's beloved.* https://ir.stonybrook.edu/xmului/handle/11401/77506

Greenwood, B., Hardeman, R., Huang, L., & Sojourner, A. (2020). Physician-patient racial concordance and disparities in birthing mortality for newborns. *Proceedings of the National Academy of Sciences, 117*(35), 21194–21200.

Hamilton, B., Martin, J. & Osterman, M. (2022, May). *Births: Provisional data for* 2021. Center for Disease Control and Prevention National Vital Statistics System #20. https://www.cdc.gov/nchs/data/vsrr/vsrr020.pdf

Hannah-Jones, N. (2021). *The 1619 Project: A new origin story.* One World.

Harper, K. (2021). *The ethos of black motherhood in America: Only white women get pregnant.* Lexington Books.

Healthy People. 2030, U.S. Department of Health and Human Services, Office of Disease Prevention and Health Promotion. https://health.gov/healthypeople/objectives-and-data/social-determinants-health

Hoffman, L., Trawalter, S., Axt, J., & Oliver, N. (2016). Racial bias in pain assessment and treatment recommendations, and false beliefs about biological differences between blacks and whites. *Proceedings of the National Academy of the United States of America, 113*(16), 4296–4301. https://doi.org/10.1073/pnas.1516047113

Howe, L., Hardebeck, E., Eberhardt, J., & Crum, A. (2020). White patient's physical responses to healthcare treatments are influenced by provider race and gender. *Psychological and Cognitive Sciences, 119*(27), e2007717119. https://doi.org/10.1075/pnas.2007717119

Hoyert, D. L. (2022). *Maternal mortality rates in the United States, 2020.* National Center for Health Statistics, health E-stats 2022. https://doi.org/10.15620/cdc:113967

Johnson, A., Kirk, R., Rosenblum, K. L., & Muzik, M. (2015). Enhancing breastfeeding rates among African American women: A systematic review of current psychosocial interventions. *Breastfeed Medicine, 10*(1), 45–62. https://doi.org/10.1089/bfm.2014.0023

Jones-Rogers, S. (2017). '[S]he could…spare one ample breast for the profit of her owner': White mothers and enslaved wet nurses'-invisible labor in American slave markets. *Slavery and Abolition, 38*(2), 337–355.

Meghani, S., Eeeseung, B., & Gallagher, R. (2012). Time to take stock: A meta-analysis and systematic review of analgesic treatment disparities for pain in the United States. *Pain Medicine, 13*(2), 150–174. https://doi.org/10.1111/j.1526-4637.2022.01310.x

Meier, P., Engstrom, J., Patel, A., Jeiger, B., & Bruns, N. (2010). Improving the use of human milk during and after the NICU stay. *Clinics in Perinatology, 37*, 217–245.

Owens, D. (2017). *Medical bondage: Race, gender, and the origins of American gynecology.* University of Georgia Press.

Patruno, P. (2015, November 26). The American dream film [video]. YouTube https://www.youtube.com/watch?v=_UCXCcTpS6c

Purser, J., Harrison, S., & Hung, P. (2022). Going the distance: Association between adverse birth outcomes and obstetric provider distances for adolescent pregnancies in South Carolina. *Journal of Rural Health, 38*(1), 171–179. https://doi.org/10.1111/jrh.12554

Roe v. Wade, 410 U.S. 113 (1973).

Rosenbaum, S. (2022). *A public health paradox: States with the strictest abortion laws have the weakest maternal and child health outcomes.* Commonwealth Fund. https://doi.org/10.26099/rn2g-3k42

Schreiber, M. (2022, May 24). Baby formula shortage highlights inequality in US maternal support. The Guardian. https://www.theguardian.com/environment/2022/may/24/baby-formula-shortage-breastfeeding-inequality?CMP=share_btn_link

Shen, M. J., Peterson, E. B., Costas-Muñiz, R., Hernandez, M. H., Jewell, S. T., Matsoukas, K., & Bylund, C. L. (2018). The effects of race and racial concordance on patient-physician communication: A systematic review of the literature. *Journal of Racial and Ethnic Health Disparities, 5*(1), 117–140.

Simmons, R. (2021). *Exploring the culture of breastfeeding education at historically black colleges and universities: Discovering institutional homogeneity of breastfeeding education.* Doctoral dissertation, the Indiana University of Pennsylvania]. ProQuest Dissertations Publishing.

Staton, L., Panda, M., Chen, I., Genao, I., Kurz, J., Pasanen, M., Mechaber, A., Menon, M., O'Rorke, J., Wood, J., Rosenberg, E., Faeslis, C., Carey, T., Calleson, D., & Cykert, S. (2007). When race matters: Disagreement in pain perception between patients and their physicians in primary care. *Journal of National Medical Association, 99*(5), 532–538.

Todd, H., Deaton, C., D'Adamo, A., & Goe, L. (2000). Ethnicity, and analgesic practice. *Annuals of Emergency Medicine, 35*(1), 11–16.

Webb, M. (2022). Black women's health imperative releases statement on supreme Court's decision to overturn roe v. Wade. https://www.prnewswire.com/news-releases/black-womens-health-imperative-releases-statement-on-supreme-courts-decision-to-overturn-roe-v-wade-301574959.html

Yehuda, R., & Lehrner, A. (2018). Intergenerational transmission of trauma effects: Putative role of epigenetic mechanisms. *World Psychiatry, 17*(3), 243–257. https://doi.org/10.1002/wps.20568

Chapter 9
Cultural Conflicts and Maternal Autonomy

Joan MacEachen

9.1 The Autonomy of American Mothers

Professional medical ethics has evolved over the past 50 years from a position of paternalism to one of respect for and fostering of patient autonomy. As initially presented in *The Principles of Biomedical Ethics* (Beauchamp & Childress, 1979), autonomy is one of the four principles of medical ethics along with beneficence, non-maleficence, and justice. Later work by Beauchamp and Childress (2019) defines autonomous decision-making as intentionality, substantial understanding, and freedom from controlling influences. In health care delivery, this process has often been interpreted as individual patient choice about acceptance of medical advice and interventions. With respect to motherhood, autonomy starts with the choice to become pregnant, to continue a pregnancy, and choices about health care during the childbearing cycle.

Although the definition of autonomy explicitly precludes controlling influences, decision-making is influenced by interpersonal relationships and the broader social environments (MacKenzie & Stoljar, 2000). This chapter examines maternal autonomy in light of the current American social environment. Most recently, conflict between maternal rights versus fetal rights has escalated in the context of polarized views on individual rights. On a more long-term basis, the American cultural value of individualism has contrasted sharply with collective identity, as exemplified by American Indian and Alaskan Native (AI/AN) population groups. Additionally, expanded social internet information has increased public knowledge about available choices of timing, place, and provider for care during childbearing. For example, internet information, in addition to product availability, has facilitated the capacity for home-based in vitro fertilization as well as pregnancy termination.

J. MacEachen (✉)
Healthcare Provider, Durango, CO, USA

© The Author(s), under exclusive license to Springer Nature Switzerland AG 2023
B. A. Anderson, L. R. Roberts (eds.), *Maternal Health and American Cultural Values*,
Global Maternal and Child Health, https://doi.org/10.1007/978-3-031-23969-4_9

High technology in the birth process has vastly impacted the context of choices. Most recently, the exposure of childbearing women to COVID-19 by the unvaccinated population and COVID-19 vaccination uptake among childbearing women have influenced maternal choice and autonomy.

9.2   Individualism and Autonomy Among American Women

The cultural value of individualism focuses on personal freedom and the autonomy of each individual, including liberty of conscience. The federal government is obliged by the Constitution and, more specifically, by the Bill of Rights, to respect the individual citizen's basic rights. Over the past 250 years, the federal legislature and Supreme Court have expanded and contracted individual's rights at both federal and state levels.

Many rights were not envisioned when the original Bill of Rights was written, but have been addressed with subsequent amendments to the Constitution. Women's rights have been addressed in a limited and piecemeal fashion, most importantly by legalizing the right to vote in the 19th Amendment. Other protections for women, such as the Equal Pay Act (EPA), have addressed gender-related wage discrepancy for equal labor. These protections have been partially effective. Since the enactment of the EPA in 1963, equality in salaries has risen from 62.3% of men's earnings in 1979 to 81.1% in 2018 (U.S. Bureau of Labor Statistics., 2019). Even so, the EPA's goal of equal pay for equal work has not yet been achieved. Further attempts to protect the rights of women, such as the Equal Rights Amendment, have not been successful.

9.2.1   Legalization and Subsequent Threats to Autonomy in Pregnancy Continuation

During the 1970s the Supreme Court broadened the applicability of the Bill of Rights to hold states to the federal standard of an implicit right to privacy. This was codified in Roe v. Wade (1973), which led to the nationwide legalization of abortion as an individual maternal right. However, legal limitations to this autonomy have grown ever since. On June 24, 2022, the Supreme Court overturned *Roe v. Wade* (Roe v. Wade, 1973). The Pew Research Center reports that 57% of Americans disapprove of this Supreme Court's decision (https://www.pewresearch.org/fact-tank/2022/07/15/key-facts-about-the-abortion- debate-in-america/).

At one extreme, some evangelical Christian groups and the Roman Catholic Church have decreed that abortion should be illegal and have been politically active in dismantling this right. The Catholic Church administers 15% of the hospitals in the USA, which are frequently the sole source of care for rural women in poverty.

The *Ethical and Religious Directives for Catholic Health Care Services, fifth edition* states "Abortion (that is, the directly intended termination of pregnancy before viability or the directly intended destruction of a viable fetus) is never permitted" (Malloy, 2009, p.26). The Catholic Church's ban on abortion care extends to fertility regulation including tubal ligation, vasectomy, and emergency contraception. This stance poses a significant restriction on the autonomy of poor, rural women.

Additionally, the Hyde amendment, passed in 1976, prohibits the use of federal funds for abortions, unless the mother's life is at risk if she were to carry the fetus to viability. Recipients of Medicaid, Medicare, the Children's Health Insurance Program, federal employees, military personnel, veterans, Native Americans, and low-income women living in the District of Columbia are denied federal funds for pregnancy termination. In 2019 this left 7.8 million low-income women aged 15–49, half of whom are women of color, with Medicaid coverage but without abortion coverage except as noted above (https://www.guttmacher.org/fact-sheet/hyde-amendment.). Of the money spent on health care in the USA, 56% is government subsidized including Medicare, Medicaid, Indian Health Services (HIS), military, and veterans (Centers for Medicare & Medicaid Services [CMMS], 2021). This funding restriction has impacted women's autonomy in that it has excluded federal funding for abortion since 1976.

Furthermore, in 2019, Title X, the federal program which supports comprehensive family planning for low-income clients, included a *gag order* in which health care providers working in clinics that received federal funds were prohibited from counseling about abortions or referring clients to abortion services. The Biden Administration has subsequently rescinded this order, but many providers of family planning services have left the Title X network and need to obtain alternate funding for clinic services (https://19thnews.org/2021/10/title-x-contraceptionfamily-planning). This leaves many women, especially those of limited economic stability, without autonomy and individual choice about their reproductive health.

The legal threats to autonomy in pregnancy continuation have gradually accelerated. In 1992 the Supreme Court case *Planned Parenthood of Southeastern Pennsylvania v. Casey,* restored power to the states to regulate abortions, as long as the states did not place legal restrictions posing undue burden for women seeking to abort a fetus before viability (Planned Parenthood of Southeastern Pennsylvania v. Casey, 1992). In 2021, Texas has enacted legislation which restricted abortion beyond six weeks of pregnancy and expands the cultural value of individualism beyond maternal rights to enabling individual citizens to act as vigilantes and to report and sue anyone, including health professionals, for assisting in an abortion beyond this designated time period (Charo, 2021). If the vigilante plaintiffs are successful, the law allows them to collect a bounty of at least $10,000 plus legal fees from those they sue. If they lose, they are not liable to pay the defendant's legal costs (https://www.nytimes.com/2021/09/10/us/politics/texas-abortion-law-facts.html). Within the first month of this new legislation in Texas, the most restrictive in the nation, abortions fell by 60% (https://www.latimes.com/world-nation/story/2022-02-11/abortions-texas-fell-first-month-new-law).

9.2.2 Social Determinants of Health and Restricted Access to Abortion Services

Restrictions to abortion access are sometimes defended as necessary for the protection of women from possible post-abortion post-traumatic stress disorder (PTSD) and the protection of fetal life. These ideas reflect the cultural conflicts surrounding the individual autonomy of American mothers. This is a dichotomy in cultural values as prevention of PTSD is not noted in many other aspects of American life, including sending young men and women into war or tolerating undermining social determinants of health (SDoH), such as childhood poverty and intimate partner violence. The real issue is the control of women's autonomy.

The limitation of women's autonomy has its roots in the former slave-holding states, which historically have had the most restrictive abortion access. According to research findings, accusations of "low morality, excessive sensuality, sexual availability and absence of maternal feeling" among emancipated slaves led to the conclusion that these women were incapable of marrying legally, maintaining a home, or educating their children (Cowling et al., 2017). The resultant longstanding racial and gender employment discrimination has generated low-wage, precarious service jobs. Dual-earner households have become a financial necessity, which has worsened the stress already felt by women who provide the unwaged labor of childrearing and homemaking. Families with single breadwinners and caretakers who turn to welfare for assistance have encountered rampant racial and gender discrimination, inadequate payments, and burdensome work requirements (Matthiesen, 2022).

Restriction of access to abortion services is linked to deteriorating SDoH, especially those linked to economic stability and education access. Conversely, women able to obtain abortions have been more likely to complete a post-secondary degree (Ralph et al., 2019). According to the Guttmacher Institute, women seeking abortions span the childbearing range (15-49 years) as well as all religions, and socioeconomic levels. Nearly one in four women has had an abortion in her lifetime, and 59% already have had one child (see https://www.guttmacher.org/video/2021/who-has-abortions-united-states-part-1). Public health studies have documented that low-income women and women of color, who comprise 75% of abortion recipients, have had much less access to abortion and subsequently face worsening SDoH (Jones et al., 2019; Wagster & Willingham, 2022, Feb 2) (see also https://www.guttmacher.org/video/2021/who-has-abortions-united-states-part-1).

A number of studies have demonstrated worsening SDoH and maternal health outcomes resulting from abortion restriction. Abortion denial increases debt load by 78% as well as bankruptcies and evictions by 81% (Miller et al., 2020). Poor physical and/or mental health, domestic violence, and economic instability, resulting in inadequate nutrition and poverty, are potential maternal health outcomes (Gerdts et al., 2016). Women with economic stability are more likely to have private health insurance or the resources to afford private abortion services and to find abortion services even in the current restricted environment. Abortion is a safe procedure that involves less risk than carrying a pregnancy to term (National Academy of Sciences,

2018; Raymond & Grimes, 2012). A recent Cochrane Review supports the conclusion that self-administration of pills for early abortion with limited involvement of health professionals has similar outcomes to medical abortion administered by professionals in health facilities (Gambir et al., 2020). There is not yet sufficient evidence to compare the risk of complications of medical abortions which require surgical intervention.

9.2.3 Social Determinants of Health and Access to Fertility Control

Despite widespread availability of contraception in the USA, the percentage of unplanned pregnancies, either unintended or unwanted, continues to be high (Guttmacher Institute, 2019). Births involving unplanned pregnancies are not necessarily unwanted by either the mother and/or her partner. However, pregnancy by surprise does have the potential to affect the SDoH impacting the whole family.

Births from unintended pregnancies can have a negative impact on the development of earlier-born children. A recent study revealed that the earlier-born children of mothers with unplanned completed pregnancy had lower mean child development scores compared to the earlier-born children of women who received a desired abortion (Foster et al., 2019). Unintended pregnancy is also associated with a higher risk of intimate partner violence (IPV) including birth control sabotage or emotional pressures by either partner for maintenance of the pregnancy or seeking an abortion (Goodwin et al., 2000; Hasstedt & Rowan, 2016). A recent study revealed that pregnant women in the USA die by homicide at more than twice the rate of other pregnancy-related causes, frequently killed by a partner. Pregnant Black women are nearly three times more likely to die of homicide than when not pregnant. Pregnant girls and women between the ages of 10 and 24 are at the highest risk of homicide (Wallace et al., 2021).

On a positive note, the proportion of pregnancies with desired timing has increased over the last decade, especially in the Western and the Midwestern states (Kost et al., 2021). This has been part of a long-term declining trend in the rate of unintended pregnancies and the proportion of women seeking abortions in the USA over the past 50 years (Finer & Zolna, 2014, 2016; Sonfield et al., 2014). The number of teen births is at a record low and the birth rate has declined among women in all races (National Center for Health Statistics, 2022). Teens and women ages 20 to 24 report having less sex and increased use of contraception, especially highly effective long-acting reversible contraception such as implants and intrauterine devices (Eeckhaut et al., 2021). Teenagers reported that they have been influenced by information on MTV depicting a hypothetical scenario about the struggles of teen mothers (Kearney, 2014). The use of emergency contraception has also increased between 2002 and 2015, from 8.2% to 22.9% (Martinez & Abma, 2020).

Likewise, older women also have had increased access to effective contraception and emergency contraception (Eeckhaut et al., 2021). Income and education influence the choice of permanent contraception, with the use of female permanent methods being more common at lower levels of income and education, while those at a higher level more frequently relied on partner vasectomy (Kavanaugh & Pliskin, 2020). Access to fertility control methods has improved over the past two decades, giving mothers more autonomy in making informed decisions about if and when to become pregnant.

9.2.4 Autonomy in Decisions about Birth Practices

Autonomy and sense of control are critical to the mental health of childbearing women. The use of a birth plan, as discussed earlier in this book, helps mothers communicate their choices to their health care providers. Some of the decisions a mother may or may not make are choice of birth attendant, place of delivery, the level of technology used in the birth process, and who accompanies the birthing woman, such as partners, family, friends, and doulas.

The cultural value of individualism around birth practices can create conflict between the mother and her health care provider. Most providers are highly respectful of a mother's autonomy and will seek to accommodate within the limits of good medical judgment (see https://www.acog.org/clinical/clinical-guidance/ committee-opinion/articles/2017/04/planned-home-birth). Much of this choice, however, has been moderated by the COVID-19 pandemic and necessary restrictions in hospitals. Although most births take place in the hospital setting, there has been an increase in planned out-of-hospital births during the COVID-19 pandemic (Gregory et al., 2021).

9.3 Exemplar: Autonomy Among American Indian and Alaska Native Mothers

The 500-year interface between the dominant American cultural value of individualism and the value of collectivism among American Indian and Alaskan Natives (AI/AN) has been a source of cultural conflict. Navajo participants in a study of the largest American Indian tribe in the USA report that while they are influenced by and value individualism, they also practice the collectivistic Navajo cultural values (Hossain et al., 2011). I (JME) have worked for 28 years as a family medicine physician and public health specialist with different tribes. I have attended births and provided care for AI/AN women representing tribes in the southwest, west, and Alaska living on rural, remote reservations. My experience is that collective identity among AI/AN continues to be strong. For example, when tribal artistry was displayed in museums, basket weavers and *beaders*, those who create exquisite pieces of art with beads and shells, hesitated to have their names attached to their individual craftsmanship. It was also evident in the ostracism of primary school students who were acknowledged for their individual achievements in school. Some scholars state that this reticence to acknowledge personal academic excellence contributes to the high school drop-out rate among Native American youth, up to three times that of the national average (Cornelius, 2002) or to feeling uncomfortable returning to their tribal reservation home after graduating from college (Kramer, 1991). Those who more strongly value individualism described their experiences to me as similar to lobsters in a pot with those closest to escaping clawed back into the pot by fellow lobsters.

This lack of comfort in dealing with the cultural value of individualism and the comfort in tribal collectivism has been reinforced by American history and by the SDoH affecting the lives of many AI/AN. I observed hesitation among many of my patients in trusting allopathic medications and procedures. In a recent study in the Midwest, 117 participants of various ethnic minorities were queried about satisfaction with their current health care providers. The perception of poor treatment predicted lower levels of satisfaction and racist experiences predicted fear of conventional health care services. The AI/AN participants reported poor treatment most frequently (Shepherd et al., 2018). Childbearing AI/AN women have reported feeling disrespected and being stereotyped as *drunks and drug users* (Heck et al., 2021).

9.3.1 Health Outcomes Among American Indian/Alaska Native Mothers

There are significant differences in maternal health outcomes among AI/AN compared to the general population. The maternal mortality rate (MMR) among AI/AN is 29.7/100,000 live births compared to the general population average at 16.7/100,000 live births (Heck et al., 2021; Petersen et al., 2019). A recent report in 2021 cites the general USA MMR at 23.8/100,000 due to COVID-19 pandemic disruptions (see https://www.nytimes.com/2022/02/23/health/maternal-deaths-pandemic.html). Maternal mortality among AI/AN mothers is almost as high as Black mothers, ranking second highest in the nation (United Health Foundation, 2021).

The three leading causes of AI/AN maternal mortality are hemorrhage (19.7%), cardiomyopathies (14.4%), and hypertensive disorders of pregnancy (12.8%) (Heck et al., 2021; Petersen et al., 2019). Postpartum hemorrhage and uterine atony are much higher among AI/AN mothers than among White mothers (Chalouhi et al., 2015), although the reasons are not well understood. Because blood transfusions carry high risks, current practice emphasizes prevention and early recognition of postpartum hemorrhage (Evensen et al., 2017). Cardiomyopathy and hypertensive disorders of pregnancy among AI/AN mothers may be partially explained by the high rate of diabetes, obesity, and hypertension. A study in Washington State examined a 17% increased risk of pre-eclampsia compared to White women, adjusted for age, socioeconomic status, and smoking. This study revealed that obesity accounts for most of the excess rate of pre-eclampsia among this population (Zamora-Kapoor et al., 2016). Initial diagnosis of hypertensive disorders during pregnancy is higher for AI/AN than for White women (12.8% and 6.7% respectively, p < 0.05) (Petersen et al., 2019). Hypertensive disorders of pregnancy are associated with pre-eclampsia as well as with cardiomyopathy (Behrens et al., 2016).

In addition to these chronic conditions, which are often exacerbated by childbearing, AI/AN women face a greater number of major stressors than women of other racial and ethnic origins in the 12 months prior to pregnancy (Whitehead et al., 2003). These stressors include high rates of IPV, rape, and a history of adverse childhood events (ACE) (Evans-Campbell et al., 2006). Alcohol abuse, tobacco use, and higher rates of suicide and homicide affect AI/AN in general as well as childbearing women as compared to other populations in the USA (Gone & Trimble, 2012; James et al., 2021). All of these factors are examples of SDoH that undermine maternal health and contribute to maternal mortality.

In Healthy People, 2030, the SDoH domain *Health Care Access and Quality* is particularly germane (Healthy People, 2030). For AI/AN mothers, especially those on rural, remote reservations where access and availability of preconceptual, childbearing, and health care across the lifespan are often limited. Historically AI/AN tribes signed treaties with the US government, ceding claims to lands and natural resources in exchange for guaranteed health care for themselves and their descendants. The Indian Health Service, an agency within the US Department of Health and Human Services, was established in 1955 to administer comprehensive health care to the 574 federally recognized tribes. Its stated purpose is to provide available and accessible health care and public health services to AI/AN. It currently provides services to 2.6 million AI/AN (see http://www.hhs.gov/healthcare/facts-and-features/fact-sheets/aca-and-american-indian-and-alaska-native-people/index.html).

IHS health care has been jeopardized by decisions in national budget appropriations and stipulations of health care coverage, although improved with the implementation of the Affordable Care Act (U.S. Department of Health and Human Services, 2021). Limited coverage contributes to less prevention and treatment of the chronic conditions, amplifying maternal mortality among AI/AN mothers. In my 28-year career with HIS, I have witnessed first-hand how the health care needs of my patients were pitted against these budget-slashing politics.

9.3.2 Examples of Collectivism as Supportive to Maternal Health

I have also witnessed how the culture of collectivism among AI/AN helps the mother in making decisions while seeking to protect her against the broader cultural conflicts facing American mothers. My respected colleague, Dr. Elise Pletnikoff, is a member of the Alaska Native tribe, the Aleut/Sun'aq. She currently practices medicine in Kodiak, Alaska where I also previously practiced. She describes how the culture of collectivism among Alaska Natives supports the autonomy and health of mothers (see Box 9.1).

Box 9.1 Interview with Elise Pletnikoff, MD, Aleut/Sun'aq tribe
The most valued relationship in the Alaska Native community is between a mother and her child, regardless of age of the child. Children are universally seen as a gift, and cared for collectively by the extended family, most often the females in the extended family. Teen pregnancies are often considered to be a positive life change, as the extended family will support the dyad through the mother's upcoming education and life changes.

Birth is seen as a physiologically normal and routine process—what it takes to get a child, and nothing to be afraid of as our ancestors did it. Pregnancy, childbirth, breastfeeding, co-sleeping, and nearly continuous baby wearing throughout the first 6–12 months are considered by the community to be healthy engagement with the next generation. Fathers are often moved to a different bedroom or sleeping space to support the maternal baby dyad during the first months or years, as a normal way for the mother to care for the baby.

The baby is immediately of the extended family, and is the expected source of pride for all generations. Grandparents and great grandparents are intimately involved in caring for babies and children, and often are central to the first experiences of sharing traditional foods with the child and supporting parents in exposing the new generation to our traditional lifestyle, such as fishing, hunting, berry picking, and food processing. Babies and children are included in all aspect of daily life, and exposed to our close relationship with the land early and as a routine part of daily life.

Alaska Native mothers typically identify their children as their primary responsibility in life. This does not exclude education and a career if the mother has a caring home environment often provided by extended family due to this intense sense of responsibility for the child. The culture supports the Alaska Native woman to be autonomous and vocal about which values are best in raising their children-acceptance of and love for the child, multigenerational support, and deep community engagement.
(Personal communication, Elise Pletnikoff, February 18, 2022).

As a primary care physician, I (JME) have attended the births of many AI/AN women surrounded by their extended family and their older children. The women had such strength and control in birthing. Family members saw to the needs of the older children. The birth of the new baby was a positive experience.

A Ute tribal tradition, grounded in collectivism, supports the new mother staying home following birth, enabling the maternal-infant bond. Grandmothers have a primary role as they care for grandchildren and transmit cultural values. Among the Apache, there is a tradition of aunts adopting an infant as their own when the mother is emotionally or physically unable to provide care. Reliance on families to care for the children does have the possibility of encouraging maternal passivity and boredom. Sometimes new mothers leave home for extended periods to seek entertainment and stimulation.

The culture of collectivism, as opposed to rugged individualism and autonomy, is a countercurrent in AI/AN populations which serves to both restrict autonomy and support maternal wellbeing. It can lead to passivity and an abrogation of maternal duties to other family members, as well as alienation from allopathic medical practices. On the other hand, it can be supportive for both mother and baby and a source of pride for the extended family. Mothers may be able to pursue formal education and a career while being confident that their children will be cared for and taught the traditional lifestyle.

9.4 Summary

Individualism is highly cherished as a cultural value among Americans. At this point in time, American women are benefitting from internet information and product availability supporting increased autonomy in decisions on when and how to bear children. However, these gains are generally available to women in higher socio-economic brackets while the choices available to those in poverty have become more limited. The most significant threat to maternal autonomy at this time is the restriction on availability of abortion. Those states with the least effective or inadequate sex education have refused Medicaid expansion to provide health care insurance to mothers and their children.

The Supreme Court reversal of *Roe v. Wade* has instituted abortion-access restrictions (Guttmacher, 2022). The burden of caring for the additional pregnancies will be borne most heavily by those living in poverty, who may not be able to travel to states where some level of abortion still is permitted. This will accelerate worsening SDoH among these women, risking complications of childbearing and facing four times greater odds of subsequently living in poverty (Ralph et al., 2019).

Political decisions are significantly influenced by the cultural value of individualism. Policy decisions based on the rights of the individual have had a significant impact on maternal health outcomes. Health care ethics have evolved from paternalism to patient autonomy, including choices on timing and continuation of pregnancy and decisions around birth practices. Freedom of information on the internet has allowed individual decision-making on at-home in-vitro fertilization, home-based abortion, and use of both long-term contraceptives, and emergency contraception.

The importance of access to information has been highlighted in the American response to COVID-19. Both information and misinformation have been highly influential in childbearing decisions. Just as it took a 50-year effort to insure voting rights to women, it will require long-term political decision-making and policy for all women, not just those of high socioeconomic status, to gain full autonomy over choices on timing and continuation of pregnancy and choices around birth practices.

References

Beauchamp, T., & Childress, J. (1979). *Principles of biomedical ethics* (1st ed.). Oxford University Press.

Beauchamp, T., & Childress, J. (2019). *Principles of biomedical ethics* (8th ed.). Oxford University Press.

Behrens, I., Basit, S., Lykke, J. A., Ranthe, M. F., Wohlfahrt, J., Bundgaard, H., Melbye, M., & Boyd, H. A. (2016). Association between hypertensive disorders of pregnancy and later risk of cardiomyopathy. *JAMA, 315*(10), 1026–1033.

Centers for Medicare & Medicaid Services. (2021, December 15). National Health Expenditure Fact Sheet. https://www.cms.gov/Research-Statistics-Data-and-Systems/Statistics-Trends-and-Reports/NationalHealthExpendData/NHE-Fact-Sheet

Chalouhi, S. E., Tarutis, J., Barros, G., Starke, R. M., & Mozurkewich, E. L. (2015). Risk of post-partum hemorrhage among native American women. *International Journal of Gynecology & Obstetrics, 131*(3), 269–272.

Charo, R. (2021). Vigilante injustice—Deputizing and weaponizing the public to stop abortions. *New England Journal of Medicine, 385*(15), 1441–1442.

Cornelius, M. (2002). An exploration of possible causes of high dropout rates in native American reservation schools. *Nebraska Anthropologist, 17*(2001–2002), 18–23. https://digitalcommons.unl.edu/nebanthro/71/

Cowling, C., Machado, M., Paton, D., & West, E. (2017). Mothering slaves: Comparative perspectives on motherhood, childlessness, and the care of children in Alantic slave societies. *Slavery & Abolition, 38*, 223–231.

Eeckhaut, M. C., Rendall, M. S., & Zvavitch, P. (2021). Women's use of long-acting reversible contraception for birth timing and birth stopping. *Demography, 58*(4), 1327–1346.

Evans-Campbell, T., Lindhorst, T., Huang, B., & Walters, K. L. (2006). Interpersonal violence in the lives of urban American Indian and Alaska native women: Implications for health, mental health, and help-seeking. *American Journal of Public Health, 96*(8), 1416–1422.

Evensen, A., Anderson, J. M., & Fontaine, P. (2017). Postpartum hemorrhage: Prevention and treatment. *American Family Physician, 95*(7), 442–449.

Finer, L., & Zolna, M. (2014). Shifts in intended and unintended pregnancies in the United States, 2001–2008. *American Journal of Public Health, 104*(Suppl 1), S43–S48. https://doi.org/10.2105/AJPH.2013.301416

Finer, L., & Zolna, M. (2016). Declines in unintended pregnancy in the United States, 2008–2011. *New England Journal of Medicine, 374*(9), 843–852. https://doi.org/10.1056/NEJMsa1506575

Foster, D. G., Raifman, S. E., Gipson, J. D., Rocca, C. H., & Biggs, M. A. (2019). Effects of carrying an unwanted pregnancy to term on women's existing children. *The Journal of Pediatrics, 205*(183–189), e181.

Gambir, K., Kim, C., Necastro, K. A., Ganatra, B., & Ngo, T. D. (2020). Self-administered versus provider-administered medical abortion. *Cochrane Database of Systematic Reviews, 3*. https://doi.org/10.1002/14651858.CD013181.pub2

Gerdts, C., Dobkin, L., Foster, D. G., & Schwarz, E. B. (2016). Side effects, physical health consequences, and mortality associated with abortion and birth after an unwanted pregnancy. *Women's Health Issues, 26*(1), 55–59.

Gone, J. P., & Trimble, J. E. (2012). American Indian and Alaska native mental health: Diverse perspectives on enduring disparities. *Annual Review of Clinical Psychology, 8*, 131–160.

Goodwin, M. M., Gazmararian, J. A., Johnson, C. H., Gilbert, B. C., Saltzman, L. E., & Group, PW. (2000). Pregnancy intendedness and physical abuse around the time of pregnancy: Findings from the pregnancy risk assessment monitoring system, 1996–1997. *Maternal and Child Health Journal, 4*(2), 85–92.

Gregory, E., Ostgerman, J., & Valenzuela, C. (2021). Changes in home births by race and Hispanic origin and state of residence of mother: United States, 2018-2019 and 2019-2020.

National Vitral Statistics Reports, 70(15), 1–9. https://www.cdc.gov/nchs/data/nvsr/nvsr70/NVSR70-15.pdf

Guttmacher Institute. (2019). Unintended pregnancy in the United States. Guttmacher Institute. https://www.guttmacher.org/fact-sheet/unintended-pregnancy-united-states

Guttmacher Institute. (2022). Roe v. Wade in peril: Our latest resources. Guttmacher institute. Retrieved March 7, 2022 from https://www.guttmacher.org/article/2021/10/26-states-are-certain-or-likely-ban-abortion-without-roe-heres-which-ones-and-why

Hasstedt, K., & Rowan, A. (2016). Understanding intimate partner violence as a sexual and reproductive health and rights issue in the United States. *Guttmacher Institute.*. https://www.guttmacher.org/gpr/2016/07/understanding-intimate-partner-violence-sexual-and-reproductive-health-and-rights-issue

Healthy People. (2030). U.S. Department of Health and Human Services, Office of Disease Prevention and Health Promotion. https://health.gov/healthypeople/objectives-and-data/social-determinants-health

Heck, J. L., Jones, E. J., Bohn, D., McCage, S., Parker, J. G., Parker, M., Pierce, S. L., & Campbell, J. (2021). Maternal mortality among American Indian/Alaska native women: A scoping review. *Journal of Women's Health, 30*(2), 220–229.

Hossain, Z., Skurky, T., Joe, J., & Hunt, T. (2011). The sense of collectivism and individualism among husbands and wives in traditional and bi-cultural Navajo families on the Navajo reservation. *Journal of Comparative Family Studies, 42*(4), 543–562.

James, R., Hesketh, M. A., Benally, T. R., Johnson, S. S., Tanner, L. R., & Means, S. V. (2021). Assessing social determinants of health in a prenatal and perinatal cultural intervention for American Indians and Alaska Natives. *International Journal of Environmental Research in Public Health, 18*(21), 11079. https://doi.org/10.3390/ijerph182111079. PMID: 34769596.

Jones, R., Witwer, E., & Jerman, J. (2019). Abortion incidence and service availability in the United States, 2017. Guttmacher Institute. Retrieved Feb 2, 2022 from https://www.guttmacher.org/report/abortion-incidence-service-availability-us-2017

Kavanaugh, M. L., & Pliskin, E. (2020). Use of contraception among reproductive-aged women in the United States, 2014 and 2016. *F&S Reports, 1*(2), 83–93.

Kearney, M. S. (2014). *MTV's "16 and Pregnant", "Teen Mom" Partly Responsible for Decrease in Teen Pregnancy* [YouTube video]. Retrieved January 24, 2022 from https://youtu.be/zgg27nPFCLs

Kost, K., Maddow-Zimet, I., & Little, A. C. (2021). Pregnancies and pregnancy desires at the state level: Estimates for 2017 and trends since 2012. Guttmacher Institute. Retrieved from https://www.guttmacher.org/report/pregnancy-desires-and-pregnancies-state-level-estimates-2017.

Kramer, B. J. (1991). Education and American Indians: The experience of the Ute Indian tribe. In M. A. Gibson & J. U. Ogbu (Eds.), *Minority status and schooling: A comparative study of immigrant and involuntary minorities* (pp. 287–307). Garland Publishing.

Mackenzie, C., & Stoljar, N. (2000). *Relational autonomy: Feminist perspectives on autonomy, agency, and the social self*. Oxford University Press.

Malloy, D. J. (2009). Ethical and religious directives for Catholic health care services. *USCCB*. https://www.usccb.org/issues-and-action/human-life-and-dignity/health-care/upload/Ethical-Religious-Directives-Catholic-Health-Care-Services-fifth-edition-2009.pdf

Martinez, G. M., & Abma, J. C. (2020). *Sexual activity and contraceptive use among teenagers aged 15–19 in the United States, 2015–2017* (p. 366). National Center for Health Statistics. Retrieved Feb 4, 2022 from https://www.cdc.gov/nchs/products/databriefs/db366.htm

Matthiesen, S. (2022). *Abortion is not a "choice" without racial justice*. The Boston Review Retrieved March 4, 2022 from https:// bostonreview.net/articles/abortion-is-not-a-choice-without-racial-justice/.

Miller, S., Wherry, L. R., & Foster, D. G. (2020). The economic consequences of being denied an abortion. https://www.nber.org/system/files/working_papers/w26662/w26662.pdf.

National Academies of Sciences, E., & Medicine. (2018). The safety and quality of abortion Care in the United States. *The National Academies Press, 10*(17226/24950).

National Center for Health Statistics, (last reviewed 2022, Feb 2). Virtal statistics online data portal. Retrieved February 5, 2022 from https://www.cdc.gov/nchs/data_access/vitalstatsonline.htm

Petersen, E. E., Davis, N. L., Goodman, D., Cox, S., Syverson, C., Seed, K., Shapiro-Mendoza, C., Callaghan, W. M., & Barfield, W. (2019). Racial/ethnic disparities in pregnancy-related deaths—United States, 2007–2016. *Morbidity and Mortality Weekly Report, 68*(35), 762.

Planned Parenthood of Southeastern Pennsylvania v. Casey, 505 U.S. 833. (1992).

Ralph, L. J., Mauldon, J., Biggs, M. A., & Foster, D. G. (2019). A prospective cohort study of the effect of receiving versus being denied an abortion on educational attainment. *Women's Health Issues, 29*(6), 455–464. https://doi.org/10.1016/j.whi.2019.09.004

Raymond, E. G., & Grimes, D. A. (2012). The comparative safety of legal induced abortion and childbirth in the United States. *Obstetrics & Gynecology, 119*(2), 215–219. https://doi.org/10.1097/AOG.0b013e31823fe923

Roe v. Wade, 410 U.S. 113 (1973).

Shepherd, S. M., Willis-Esqueda, C., Paradies, Y., Sivasubramaniam, D., Sherwood, J., & Brockie, T. (2018). Racial and cultural minority experiences and perceptions of health care provision in a mid-western region. *International Journal for Equity in Health, 17*(1), 1–10.

Sonfield, A, Hasstedt, K., & Gold, R. (2014). *Moving Forward: Family Planning in the Era of Health Reform*, Guttmacher Institute. Retrieved Feb 5, 2022 from https://www.guttmacher.org/report/moving-forward-family-planning-era-health-reform

U.S. Bureau of Labor Statistics. (2019). Women in the labor force: A databook (BLS reports, Issue. U.S. Bureau of Labor Statistics https://www.bls.gov/opub/reports/womens-databook/2019/pdf/home.pdf.

U.S. Department of Health and Human Services. (2021, July 22). Health Insurance Coverage and Access to Care for American Indians and Alaska Natives: Current Trends and Key Challenges. Office of Health Policy Issue Brief HP-2021-18. Retrieved Feb 5, 2021 from https://aspe.hhs.gov/sites/default/files/2021-07/aspe-aian-health-insurance-coverage-ib.pdf

United Health Foundation. (2021). America's health rankings: Health of women and children. *United Health Foundation.*. https://www.americashealthrankings.org/explore/health-of-women-and-children/measure/maternal_mortality/state/ALL

Wagster, E. & Willingham, L. (2022, Feb 2). *Minorities bear brunt of limits on abortion.* Los Angeles Times, p. A-2 Retrieved from https://enewspaper.latimes.com/desktop/latimes/default.aspx?token=42e23962a5d74614be16bae3d62d13e7&utm_id=47693&sfmc_id=1568448&edid=84acfd92-e620-4b2b-99ae-ce7bf2a5cb8b

Wallace, M., Gillispie-Bell, V., Cruz, K., Davis, K., & Vilda, D. (2021). Homicide during pregnancy and the postpartum pPeriod in the United States, 2018–2019. *Obstetrics & Gynecology, 138*(5), 762–769.

Whitehead, N., Brogan, D., Blackmore-Prince, C., & Hill, H. (2003). Correlates of experiencing life events just before or during pregnancy. *Journal of Psychosomatic Obstetrics and Gynecology, 24*(2), 77–86.

Zamora-Kapoor, A., Nelson, L. A., Buchwald, D. S., Walker, L. R., & Mueller, B. A. (2016). Pre-eclampsia in American Indians/Alaska natives and whites: The significance of body mass index. *Maternal and Child Health Journal, 20*(11), 2233–2238.

Chapter 10
The National Conversation on Maternal Health

Barbara A. Anderson

10.1 Information Dissemination on Maternal Health

In 2010, with an update in 2011, Amnesty International released the report, *Deadly delivery: The Maternal Health Care Crisis in the USA* (Amnesty International, 2011). This report sent shock waves across the nation, documenting that 50–60% of maternal deaths in the USA are not only preventable but also related to inconsistent management of obstetrical emergencies, fragmentation in the healthcare system, inadequate health literacy among the population, increasing co-morbidity among childbearing women, and inadequate data retrieval, management, and reporting. It linked maternal health outcomes with the social determinants of health (SDoH), in particular, racism, poverty, and access to care. Scientific research and publications corroborated these findings (American College of Obstetricians and Gynecologists, 2014; Building U.S. Capacity to Review and Prevent Maternal Deaths, 2018; Creanga, 2018; Lazariu et al., 2017; MacDorman et al., 2016; Zuckerwise & Lipkind, 2017).

The Amnesty International report is an example of how the media captures and shapes public discourse beyond scholarship. The professional literature is generally evidence-based and well-presented in professional books and journals, reaching closed professional circles. It offers strategies to enhance professional performance and aims to translate research into practice through dissemination strategies (Agency for Healthcare Research Quality, 2012; Ordoñez & Serrat, 2017). It aims to link health issues with social conditions. A relatively recent publication, *Population Health and the Future of Healthcare* (Thomas, 2021), is an excellent example. It provides an analysis of links between health and the SDoH (Healthy People, 2030) through the classic journalism questions: *who, what, when, where, and how much.*

B. A. Anderson (✉)
Frontier Nursing University, Versailles, KY, USA

© The Author(s), under exclusive license to Springer Nature Switzerland AG 2023   117
B. A. Anderson, L. R. Roberts (eds.), *Maternal Health and American Cultural Values*,
Global Maternal and Child Health, https://doi.org/10.1007/978-3-031-23969-4_10

While highly valuable scholarly endeavors advance knowledge, they may be obtuse to many persons and they do not necessarily reach nor grab the attention of the nation like the Amnesty International report did. Nor do they answer the question *why?* Why, beyond the social determinants, does the nation have such shocking maternal health outcomes? That is the work of journalism as well as scholarship.

Most Americans had no idea (many still do not) that maternal mortality and morbidity in the USA is the worst among high-resource nations and frequently worse than many mid-level countries. The Amnesty report powerfully told this story, not just through facts, but also through stories. It consistently portrayed experiences and photography depicting mothers, newborns, and families affected by maternal death and poor maternal health outcomes (Amnesty International, 2011). It drove home the message of the maternal health crisis in the nation.

Storytelling is a powerful tool to translate evidence-based but disembodied facts, into the realities facing mothers, families, and healthcare providers. It is a compelling way to attract attention to an idea, to shape public opinion, to focus activism, and to support the steps in policy development (Davidson, 2017). Barrett et al. describe the use of storytelling as a key strategy in framing ethics in public health (2022). Documentaries, media interviews, podcasts, blogs, social media sites, and graphic medicine cartoons use storytelling as a powerful journalistic approach. Graphic medicine is an example of the juxtaposition between cartoon storytelling and evidence-based scholarship that promotes dissemination of information. In their recent publication, *Infertility Comics and Graphic Medicine,* Murali and Venkatesan (2022) use the medium of comics to merge scientific knowledge with messages on gender roles and infertility.

Now, over a decade after the Amnesty International report, media messages about health outcomes among American mothers are highly prevalent. They have and are shaping the national conversation. They have been influential in disseminating knowledge and providing a clarion call for better policy across the nation. This chapter focuses on media messages about maternal health outcomes in the USA, in particular maternal demographics, SDoH, and how these messages influence the national conversation.

10.2   Individualism and the Rhetoric on Maternal Health

While many media messages describe maternal health outcomes in terms of *who, what, when, where, and how much*, some go beyond to explore *why*. The premise of this book is that there are clues to the *why* in the deeply rooted American cultural values. This chapter examines one key American cultural value—*individualism*—and how this value serves to drive the national conversation.

In her work *Forget Having It All*, journalist Amy Westervelt reflects on how motherhood in America is deeply enmeshed with cultural values: "Ideas about motherhood are inextricably linked to cultural values, which is why we need to treat motherhood rhetoric as the powerful force that it is" (Westervelt, 2018, p.5).

Rhetoric is a powerful mirror of the culture. Writer Richard Rodriguez, in a themed interview titled *Imaging Others* with television journalist Bill Moyer, stated: "What America gives the world is an *I* - I, the individual" (Rodriguez, 1990, p. 85).

The cultural value of individualism is strong, pervasive, and supportive to the explanatory model of American culture. It is formative in defining American motherhood. Yet, this value of individualism is not necessarily embodied as a force of power for the mother alone. As examined in Chap. 9, the concept of individualism in maternal health decision-making may also be applied to the individual rights of others in making decisions about her reproductive choices and autonomy. The rhetoric of motherhood in the contemporary national conversation is highly focused on individual rights (and not necessarily the mother's individual rights) and conflicts between autonomy and conformity. This rhetoric drives the national conversation, reflecting a polarized and divided nation. This point has been most salient in the ruling by the Supreme Court on June 24, 2022 ruling overturning Roe v. Wade on abortion rights (see https://www.supremecourt.gov/opinions/21pdf/19-1392_6j37. pdf). This explosive decision has polarized the nation raising questions about the role of Supreme Court versus public debate and elections on a topic that has wide support by the American public. The bias of Supreme Court justices toward personal values in deciding constitutional law has been challenged prior to this current ruling (Segall, 2012).

10.2.1   Individualism and Polarization

A recent study from the Pew Research Center by Silver et al. (2021, Oct 13) revealed that while 86% of the USA population embrace the value of diversity, 59% do not agree on basic facts and 90% state there are strong tensions along political party lines. Discrimination based on race and ethnicity is acknowledged as a serious problem among 74% of the population surveyed, with those 49 years or younger viewing this in more alarming terms. The American population surveyed demonstrated the highest level of divisiveness compared to 17 other nations. According to journalist David Lauter, polarization drives the conversation (2021a, b, Oct 25) and generates a high level of political engagement and voting (Lauter, 2021a, b, Oct 18). He states that the concern is the threat to democracy if ethnic, racial, or religious conflicts escalate (2021, Oct 18).

Polarization is an expression of individualism but also a kind of conformity, according to scholars and journalists Packer and Van Bavel (2021, Nov 15). In a column titled, *Maybe the pandemic 'freethinkers' are really sheep*, they recount the historical work of French scholar, Alexis de Tocqueville, in *Democracy in America*, noting the American paradox of expressed individualism and a strong tendency to conform and be joiners. He wrote incisive observations on Benjamin Franklin's analysis of American values (2003, orig 1835, 1840). Packer and Van Bavel state, "This counterintuitive pattern might appear surprising. But it occurs because the more individualized and specialized our roles, the more dependent we become on other people to function effectively" (2021, Nov 15, p. A-13). They state that our collective strength of interdependence serves to strengthen and allow our individuality (2021, Nov 15). This concept of interlinked independence and interdependence parallels the world view on maternal autonomy among American Indians/Alaska Natives (AI/AN) as discussed in Chap. 9.

10.2.2   Language in a Divided Nation

In a recent book, titled *Language as a Social Determinant of Health*, Fererici (2022) explores how rhetoric shapes the message. Through the lens of the COVID-19 pandemic information dissemination, this edited volume has authors from around the globe comparing translation and interpretation of messages. The framework for this work has applicability for examining the dissemination of messages about maternal health outcomes in the USA. Although primarily English-speaking, the USA population experiences and often speaks languages from the far corners of the world. New York City, *Big Apple*, has more linguistic diversity than any other city in the world. Los Angeles, *City of the Angels*, comes in second. (see https://www.mapsofworld.com/answers/world/city-speaks-languages/#).

Beyond spoken languages are the diverse cultural discourses that shape world view, values, and beliefs. Within this potpourri is the cherished American cultural value of individualism, albeit expressed in many different ways. Thus there are tensions, divisions, and polarized views. Working out our differences has been widely valued. The current milieu in the USA, as tracked in the Pew Report and described by Silver et al. (2021, Oct 13), demonstrates the inherent difficulties. Divisions are rife. High disagreement on basic facts are coupled with strong political tensions. As explained by Fererici (2022) and exemplified in the daily media, the rhetoric is important. Words such as *credibility, trust, reliability, safety,* and *risk* convey deeply evocative meaning. They can convey information, but just as easily they can convey misinformation and disinformation. The national conversation on maternal health demonstrates all of these approaches with strong expressions of individual rights in decision-making.

10.2.3   Information, Misinformation, and Disinformation

Healthcare information, in the sense of being foundational for informed decision-making and essential to individualism, needs to be accurate and evidence-based from credible scientific sources, free of bias and conflicts of interest, and comprehensible to the decision-maker. Inadequate health literacy and the lack of literacy in general obstruct this process. Increasingly, publishers, content review bodies (such as Cochrane Reviews), and journal editors ask writers to provide, in addition to the original scholarly material, succinct and clear summaries of information through multiple, open-access venues. Examples are short plain-language summaries, short media presentations, and trailers to video work. In everyday parlance, these are known as the "elevator speeches," explaining the significance of the work.

Misinformation and disinformation obstruct information. Misinformation spreads false information, though not necessarily with intent to deceive (see https://www.dictionary.com/browse/misinformation). A common experience is the necessity to backtrack on an incorrect statement spoken inadvertently: "I misspoke. That is not what I meant to say." This does not define culpability or malice. Weaponizing information is disinformation. It employs deliberate falsification, manipulation of information, or spreading misinformation knowing that it is incorrect (see https://www.dictionary.com/e/misinformation-vs-disinformation-get-informed-on-the-difference/). These terms have taken on great significance as cultural conflicts have escalated in the USA.

The World Health Organization (WHO) has responded to widespread global misinformation and some disinformation by providing open access strategies and training to help healthcare providers and educators address the "infodemic." Various ways to counter the pandemic of confusion and inaccuracies in information dissemination are offered in online, self-paced learning modules (see https://openwho.org/courses/infodemic-management-101). Interactive and self-paced learning is timely with the global COVID-19 pandemic but not exclusively targeted to this topic.

On July 15, 2021, Dr. Vivek Murthy issued a press release from the Office of the Surgeon General, warning the public about the risk of significant harm through misinformation. The Surgeon General described the dangers of misinformation including the finding that social media platforms (SMP) were 70% more likely to post misinformation than accurate information (see https://www.hhs.gov/about/news/2021/07/15/us-surgeon-general-issues-advisory-during-covid-19-vaccination-push-warning-american.html). In a report in *Science*, Vosoughi et al. (2018, March 9) presented the findings on 126,000 rumors spread by greater than three million persons on Twitter from 2006 to 2017. They found that false news diffused faster than truth and reached more viewers with humans and robots equally likely to disseminate false news. Thus the impact of "alternative facts!" Understanding the risks of misinformation and the tactics of disinformation in the media is essential to guarding the health of the public (Calo, et al., 2021, Dec 8). As philosopher George Bernard Shaw is alleged to have said many years ago, "Beware of false knowledge; it is more dangerous than ignorance" (see https://www.brainyquote.com/quotes/george_bernard_shaw_141483).

While acknowledging the First Amendment right to freedom of speech, that line has been crossed in the misogyny, misinformation, and disinformation targeted toward women in the media. Maria Marron's book, *Misogyny and Media in the Age of Trump* (2020) evaluates widespread media postings denigrating women during the Trump campaign and administration. In 2018, Amnesty International released its report *Toxic Twitter: Violence and Abuse Against Women Online* which documented the human rights violations and misogyny on the SMP Twitter (Amnesty International, 2018a). Amnesty International noted that fear-inducing experiences on this SMP limited autonomy, normalized misogyny, and silenced women's voices.

Individualism was being squashed. To date, according to Amnesty International, Twitter has not mounted an effective campaign to counter this online violence (Amnesty International, 2018a, para 5).

In 2020, the United Nations Educational, Scientific, and Cultural Organization (UNESCO) and the International Center of Journalists (ICFJ) published a global study titled *Online violence against women journalists* (Posetti et al., 2020). This study demonstrated significant misogyny, misinformation, and disinformation targeted toward female journalists with 73% having experienced online violence including threats of physical and sexual violence against them or their families. Among these journalists, 20% experienced an offline live attack or abuse. Facebook was identified as the SMP with the highest number of postings threatening female journalists (Posetti et al., 2020).

Cartoon media has been specifically used to depict women unfavorably (Bland, 2020). As an example of misogynistic disinformation, the political cartoon by Angelo Lopez titled "Female journalists and online Duterte trolls" published in *Philippines Today* (2018, Nov 21) was cited in an Amnesty International report (2018b) demonstrating online abuse of women on the SMP Twitter. This cartoon called out female journalists as "pressitute," a play on the words journalism and prostitute. Amnesty International and Element AI, a global artificial intelligence company, analyzed millions of tweets, noting that Black, Latinx, Asian, and mixed-race women were 34% more likely to be targeted for this abuse than White women (Amnesty International, 2018b).

Alternative facts do matter and do cause harm. Likewise, media messages about motherhood and social concepts of "fitness" for motherhood have been and are subjected to misinformation, disinformation, racism, and additional forms of "othering." While many of the media reports on maternal health outcomes have served to spotlight the issue and encourage activism toward solutions, other reports have further ground in stereotypes about motherhood in America. Kimberly Harper points out this issue in her book, *The Ethos of Black Motherhood in America: Only White Women get Pregnant* (2020).

10.3   Motherhood According to the Media

The media is a formidable driver of the national conversation on contemporary life in America including the state of health and childbearing outcomes among American women. These messages are frequently couched within specific and marginalized demographics, e.g., minorities, those at the edges of reproductive capacity (adolescent and older age mothers), single women even if partnered, LGBTQ+ persons, mothers working outside of the home, disabled, substance-abusing, or incarcerated mothers. The conversation often revolves around the SDoH impacting these women, their fitness for motherhood, and their ability to demonstrate the American cultural value of individualism in countering stressful life events. While some of the messages are strongly supportive and empowering, others leave lingering doubts and reinforce stereotypes about the role of motherhood in America.

10.3.1 Conformity

The paradox of the American cultural value of individualism is the tendency to conform, as described in 1835 by French scholar Alexis de Tocqueville (2003, orig 1835, 1849). This paradox is evidenced in media messages about motherhood. Being a successful mother is a socially constructed concept that has an American cultural and stereotypic landscape reaching back into American history and currently grounded in the ethos of the 1950s (Doyle, 2018; Hays, 1996; Tenety, 2021, para 3). There is the expectation of enormous maternal expenditure of energy, time, and emotional investment in childrearing with lessened expectations on fathers, except for financial support. Single and working mothers are expected to conform to this stereotype of intensive mothering with further expectation of complete or partial financial support as well (Gross, 2018; Hays, 1996). Current surveys suggest that American mothers are expected to engage in intensive childrearing despite heavy expectation to simultaneously contribute to financial support and family management around the stresses of the COVID-19 pandemic (Carlson et al., 2021; Geiger et al., 2019; Miller, 2020, Nov 17). Concurrently, there is substantial literature on the increase in heavy alcohol use among mothers (Pollard et al., 2020). The "wine mom" discourse is the national conversation in which heavy alcohol use by mothers is normalized to achieve respite from messages of failure to either conform to expectations of or achieve intensive mothering (Newman & Nelson, 2021).

The media frequently report inconsistencies on what constitutes good motherhood, enough intensive mothering, or conformity to traditional gender roles for American mothers (Gross, 2018). The cultural conflict of individualism versus conformity plays out in the lives of American mothers as their right to express autonomy is subjected to polarized thinking and cultural crossfire. The expectations to conform to stereotypes of motherhood, as depicted in the 1950s, and the struggle for individualism and autonomy are witnessed in all types of journalism. National Public Radio often conducts interviews around these stereotypes. Television, documentaries, media interviews, podcasts, blogs, social media sites, popular magazines, online and print newspapers provide numerous examples.

Consultants Nate and Kaley Klemp, authors of *The 80/80 Marriage: A New Model for a Happier, Stronger Relationship,* explore the principle of fairness in domestic relationships and parenting (2021a, b). They also published a media column describing their research from in-depth interviewing of both heterosexual and same sex couples as they attempted to run households and parents during the COVID-19 pandemic. They examine the dichotomy between the 1950s stereotypes and how households are run today, factoring in the perceived stress of COVID-19. Their column, titled "A new normal for housework," points out, despite Pew Report findings of verbalized gender equality, a sense of unfairness exists in many relationships that creates tensions about gender roles, division of labor, and parenting. This finding is especially robust if roles are defined according to the 1950s model. Women are more likely to be expected to exit the workplace than men for parenting and to assume the largest portion of domestic responsibilities. They describe role confusions and conflicts over autonomy and fairness (Klemp & Klemp, 2021a, b, Nov 11). This is an exemplar of the media addressing the conflict between the cultural value of individualism and the social expectation of conformity around motherhood.

The cultural conflict between individualism and limited autonomy is highlighted in a media piece by journalist Jackie Calmes. She reports on the experiences of women testifying in accusations of sexual harassment and abuse. These women reported feeling pressure during testimony to conform to a meek, gendered role (Calmes, 2021, Aug 13). Journalist Rachel Cargle describes feeling pressures to limited personal autonomy and to conform to social expectations of childbearing. She experienced verbal accusations of selfishness when she has explained why she wishes to be child-free (Cargle, 2022, June 18). In a recent Time Magazine essay, journalist Katie Gutierrez describes her personal experience with perceived loss of autonomy and a sense of failure as she faced incredible stresses related to expectations for intensive mothering during the pandemic (2022, June 20).

An egregious example was presented in an editorial in the Los Angeles Times which explored the case of a substance-abusing young woman in Oklahoma accused of self-inducing a second-trimester abortion and arrested for murder. She was accused of being non-compliant with the abortion ban in Oklahoma (*Los Angeles Times* Editorial, 2021, Oct 22). She was exonerated of the accusation and released, but this case demonstrates a clear cultural conflict regarding autonomy. Perhaps more than any other maternal health topic, the media reports the national conversation on abortion which places maternal individualism in sharp contrast to expectations of social conformity and decision-making. Such conversations are not likely to occur around the choice of having other personally private medical procedures, e.g., deciding whether or not to have a colonoscopy. See Box 10.1 for selected media examples.

Box 10.1 National Conversation Prior to Supreme Court Overturning Roe v. Wade

POLICY AND LAW

> Associated Press. (2022a. April 22). *Judge temporarily blocks Kentucky abortion ban.* LATimes.com, p. A-7.
> Associated Press (2022b, Feb 15). *Maryland aims to protect abortion rights.* LATimes.com. p. A-7.
> Weber, P. & Associated Press. (2022, Feb 11). *Abortions in Texas fell 60% in the first month under restrictive new law.* LATimes.com. para 1. https://www.latimes.com/world-nation/story/2022-02-11/abortions-texas-fell-first-month-new-law).

HEALTHCARE WORKFORCE

> Tanner, L (2022, April 21). *Abortion training scarce, and in decline.* LATimes.com. p. A-2.

(Continued)

Box 10.1 (continued)

IMPACT ON MOTHERS

> Abrams, A. (2021, Nov 22). *On the line: Mississippi's last abortion clinic has faced court battles before, but this time it's different.* Time Magazine, pp. 34--38 with reporting from journalists Mariah Espada, Washington, D.C. and Leslie Dickstein, New York.
> King, E. (2021, Nov 12). *Abortion bans hit military women hard.* LATimes.com., p. A-11.
> Wagster, E. & Willingham, L. (2022, Feb 2) *Minorities bear brunt of limits on abortion.* LA Times.com, p. A-2.
> Wire. S. (2021, Sept 18). *How willing are taxpayers to foot bill for child care?* LATimes.com, p. A-2

10.3.2 Deviance

Mothers in America have traditionally been depicted as White, middle or upper-class married women, marginalizing mothers outside of this defined parameter. Mothers who do not fit this may be considered deviant and are subject to increased social scrutiny (Doyle, 2018; Williams, 2021). In general, mothers are blamed when families experience dysfunction, yet even more so if they do not fit the stereotypic profile (Hays, 1996; Kumar, 2020; Margolis, 2000; Vandenberg-Daves, 2014). The issue of blame is well described in an article by *Nature* editor, Anna Nowogrodzki (2021, Nov 11). While the focus of the article is the epigenetics of inherited trauma, it makes the point that the evidence is weak. Rather, it is normative culture that holds mothers accountable for adverse family outcomes. Certainly this puts an additional and potentially unfair burden on mothers, especially those struggling under imposed stereotypes. The media is mixed in blaming and supporting mothers who experience dysfunction in their families.

10.3.2.1 "Absent Mothers": The Media Profile

While two-income families are now the norm for financial survival in contemporary America, the expectation for social conformity with intensive mothering continues (Hays, 1996; Margolis, 2000; Regev, 2015, Jan 15; Vandenberg-Daves, 2014). Journalists frequently report on this issue (Matthiesen, S. (2022, Jan 25) as well as the crux of finding and affording child care (Wire, S. (2021, Sept 18). As mothers spend more time in the formal economy (Geiger et al., 2019), the "motherhood penalty" may be leveraged; the discrimination against mothers in the workplace and messages implying poor quality mothering. Paradoxically, professional success may accord greater social status than culturally defined successful motherhood. Women juggle multiple roles, sometimes at the expense of the expected cultural role of motherhood (Hays, 1996; Kumar, 2020; Margolis, 2000; Vandenberg-Daves, 2014). The media has tracked this sociological pattern and documented mothers' perceived loss of autonomy, the phenomenon of the "second shift," and the frequent occurrence of post-partum depression among American mothers. Workplace-related demands enhance that stress (Herbert, 2021, Oct 5). Among the frequent and saddest reports are the sequelae of untreated or unrecognized mental illness and post-partum depression which can result in maternal suicide and/or infant homicide. While there is ample research on the topic (Beck, 2002; Liu & Tronick, 2014; Weeks et al., 2022), almost daily, media recounts these tragic events seemingly with surprise and outrage.

The ultimate in the "absent mother" are mothers who are incarcerated or neglectful of their children due to substance abuse. Society does not cut these mothers much slack, as described in Carolyn Sufrin's book, *Jailcare: Finding the Safety Net for Women behind Bars* (2017). Criminal intent is frequently alleged. The alleged murder case in Oklahoma describes this phenomenon of blame (Los Angeles Editorial, 2021, Oct 22). Media also examines the inconsistencies and lack of evidence for "tough on crime" policies that promise greater protection for the general population against deviant mothers (Garcetto, Reiner and Krinsky, 2021, Oct 25).

10.3.2.2 "Non-traditional Mothers": Media Conversations

Non-traditional mothers, such as single mothers or partnered couples outside of legal marriage, have been stigmatized for not conforming to the traditional image of the family (Sawhill et al., 2010). Recently, having children as a single parent or in a partnered relationship outside of legal marriage has gained more social acceptance. LBGQT+ persons frequently choose parenthood and marriage, now a legal path in many parts of the USA. Still, there has always been stigma against those not conforming with the stereotypic 1950s image of the family.

Single mothers are often portrayed as creating unstable or fragile families that may require rescue by the larger society (Sawhill et al., 2010). Their "fitness for motherhood" may be questioned with messages about being unpartnered, too young, too old, not heterosexual, disabled, or a person of color. If they require any level of public assistance they may be deemed out of compliance with the cultural value of individualism and labeled as welfare queens (Aquilino, 1996; Cassese & Barnes, 2019). If there is not an active two-parent heterosexual legal union, the single mother may be informed that she does not have a "real" family or may receive unsolicited and often condescending advice on both autonomy and conformity. I (BA) have been the recipient of these messages. Men who are single parents may also experience similar messages, as did my husband before we became a "blended family." These stereotypes, myths, and messages have been explored by journalists (Regev, 2015, Jan. 15).

10.3.3 *"Fitness for Motherhood"*

Who is "fit" to be a mother? Those who do not fit the traditional stereotype may be considered "imperfect." Mothers experiencing obesity, poverty, or advanced age may be subjected to increased social scrutiny, as described above (Doyle, 2018; Williams, 2021). They are often the mothers who are struggling with the most difficult SDoH, such as economic instability, unstable or inadequate housing, racism, lack of education, poverty, and low-paying employment (Cassese & Barnes, 2019; Doyle, 2018; Harper, 2020; Matthiesen, 2022; Williams, 2021). Historical messages about "fitness" for motherhood, especially about Black mothers, have embodied destructive stereotypes that persist today (Cowling et al., 2017). Media messages about the diversity of women who become mothers may be very informative and supportive in overcoming these stereotypes. They may affirm the efforts of mothers to provide protection and care, such as a recent piece by journalist Marissa Evans titled *Breast milk as COVID fighter.* This media report embedded evidenced-based research from the American Academy of Pediatrics on high COVID-19 antibody concentrations among breastfed infants of vaccinated mothers as well as stories from mothers of various ethnicities on how breastfeeding was their way of protecting their infants during the pandemic (Evans, 2021, Nov 2). Other media messages, however, may promote stereotypes, misinformation, disinformation, racism, and various forms of "othering." Some exemplars of media portrayal about fitness for motherhood are discussed below.

10.3.3.1 Disability and Fitness for Motherhood

Disabled women may experience very hurtful stereotypes about fitness. Rebekah Taussig, mother, teacher, journalist, cancer-survivor, and wheelchair-bound paraplegic, describes these experiences in her work, *Sitting Pretty: The View from my Ordinary Resilient Disabled Body* (2020). After her son was born, she describes venturing out to her baby's first medical appointment in an excellent piece published in *Time Magazine* (Taussig, 2021, April 28). Her reflections on othering, mistrust, and social scrutiny as a disabled mother reached audiences across the globe, helping to dispel misinformation. Journalist Sonja Sharp researched and published a stunning in-depth report on the issues of fitness for disabled mothers. As the awardee of the 2021 University of Southern California Annenberg Center for Health Journalist Fellowship, her journalism was comprehensive, covering a range of disabling conditions, responses by both fearful and supportive healthcare providers, social responses experienced by childbearing disabled mothers, and poignant stories of disabled mothers including childbearing disabled healthcare providers (Sharp, 2021, Oct 3). Sharp uses storytelling as a powerful tool to convey information and dispel misinformation.

This journalist describes how disabled mothers receive many messages about lack of fitness for their role as mothers. They may be discouraged from bearing, adopting, raising, or retaining custody of children. They are more likely to lose their children in a custody battle than most women and they may be encouraged or even expected to terminate a desired pregnancy. They may have difficulty obtaining adequate and standard maternity care. Based upon their disability, they are more likely to be pressured into operative delivery procedures that are not evidence-based. Their fitness is often questioned, even by strangers, who register surprise that disabled persons have reproductive organs, can engage in sexual activities, desire children, and are capable of childrearing (Sharp, 2021, Oct 3).

I (BA) have done a great deal of health education with disabled women, many who desired to become mothers. The following is a composite story of the many women I have worked with: A traumatically injured paraplegic woman and her fiancé asked me these questions: Would they be able to have a family? What was the best method of contraception to use until they were ready to start a family? What social barriers might they experience when a mother is disabled? In addition, were the usual questions that young couples have about pregnancy, birth, and childcare. We launched into long and thoughtful discussions. One day a physician from another medical specialty walked into our session (uninvited) while I was talking with the couple. He asked me why I was spending so much time counseling this disabled woman about reproduction. The woman and her fiancé were shocked (as was I). The young man responded in anger, "We asked her to teach us about having a family and this is part of what we need to know about my fiancée's self-care. And, by the way, we do plan to have a family and you were not invited into this meeting with our health educator." Flustered, the physician left. Later, I sought out the "uninvited" healthcare provider to discuss this incident. He graciously admitted that he had learned a lot from that encounter. Later, we all went to the wedding—this time he laughingly noted he was "invited." A lovely child arrived a year later, followed by two more perfect babies. The couple made the accommodations necessary, not conforming to stereotypic messages but focusing on the autonomy of their lives.

10.3.3.2   Race, Ethnicity, and Fitness for Motherhood

Language can be a SDoH. Words can be inclusive or they can convey stereotypes. Some words have especially strong evocative meaning around motherhood: *credibility, trust, reliability, safety, and risk.* They can provide accurate information from which to make informed and autonomous decisions, encourage program and policy development, and promote social inclusiveness. Conversely, words can also skew the conversation or be weaponized to deliver disinformation. The national conversation on maternal health outcomes demonstrates accurate information, misinformation, and disinformation on fitness for motherhood. It confronts and reflects culturally polarized views on who has the right to make decisions about motherhood and who is fit to be a mother, often couched in terms of ethnicity and race.

Mothers who face adverse outcomes related to childbearing, substance abuse challenges, and violence are frequently described in the media in terms of race and ethnicity. Other SDoH are often ignored, as exemplified in some recent media pieces. When media reports on AI/AN women, it is often in the context of the violence these mothers face. Deron Marquez, co-founder of the Tribal Administration Program at Claremont Graduate University, and his colleagues recently published an excellent media piece on the high rate of violence against AI/AN women (Marquez, Marquez & Gover, 2021, Nov 10). Their article, entitled *Indigenous Women Face Egregious Harm,* describes this important cause of mortality among AI/AN mothers (2021, Nov 10). Journalist Audrey McAvoy (2021, Oct 9) reported from Hawaii on violence against Native Hawaiian women. She makes the point that the national conversation often sidelines the issues faced by Native Hawaiian women because they are not included in the Indian Health Service (IHS). Other causes of maternal death and morbidity among AI/AN often fall off the media radar. I have listened to some deep anger among Native women and their healthcare providers about the laser focus of the media on Black maternal mortality, while neglecting the almost comparable maternal mortality among AI/AN mothers.

The media depicts many facets of threats to maternal health including violence, drugs, and mental health issues. In a recent article in *Nature*, homicide, as a leading cause of maternal death, was explored by journalist Nidhi Subbaraman (2021, Nov 25). A superb, well-balanced article, although the compelling photograph in the article featured Black women, despite this being an issue across all ethnicities. Another piece by Friedman and Hansen, who are healthcare providers and addiction specialists, examined substance abuse deaths as a racial justice issue (2021, Nov 23). It described the shifting trend in drug-related deaths from Whites to "communities of color," primarily focusing on Blacks living in large metro areas. It also described the trend away from White deaths caused by prescription opioids to Black deaths (Native Americans were mentioned once) due to lack of "harm reduction" (not defined), incarceration, and poor post-prison social networks. Not disputing the myriad of SDoH at play here, the point is that Whites were portrayed as dying from overdoses of legal drugs prior to more control of addictive prescription drugs. Overdose deaths among Blacks (and communities of color) were linked to criminality. Regardless of intent to call for social justice and decriminalizing drugs, the message was clear: This is a problem primarily of Blacks and it is linked to criminality.

Kimberly Harper (2020) in her book titled *The Ethos of Black Motherhood in America: Only White Women get Pregnant* describes the social designation of fitness for motherhood, per the traditional 1950s ideal, as marginalizing mothers who do not fit this pattern. She explores cultural messages that denigrate mothers who do not fit this cultural ideal. Such messages reinforce stereotypes. A recent article by journalists Walker and Boling (2022) reports findings from semi-structured interviews with four women journalists who reported on Black maternal mortality. Six themes emerged in this qualitative study:

- Implications of inclusion of racial profiles in reporting
- Need for nuanced coverage
- Role of advocacy among journalists
- Complications of reporting on race issues

- Importance of citing persons of color in reports
- The influence of celebrities in coverage (Walker & Boling, 2022).

They emphasized the need for balanced and continual media advocacy in the national conversation about Black maternal mortality. They also reflected upon journalism norms that may encourage inappropriate citing of sources and diluting of the extent and depth of the issue (Walker and Boling, 2022). This work points to the importance of journalism in crafting messages that not only accurately report issues but also reframe the narrative toward social justice.

Many times in my clinical experience as a nurse-midwife, I have heard healthcare providers and staff describe substance-abusing mothers as follows, "This mother who has a substance use problem" (a White patient) or "That Black woman who is drug-addicted and pregnant" (a Black patient). Herein lies not only implicit racial bias but explicit discrimination. The White patient was first described as a mother, using the adjective "this" (closer proximity) and classifying her as a mother, followed by delineating a potential problem she was experiencing. The Black patient, using the distancing adjective "that," linked with her race, makes this the primary identifier. Then she was described as a woman, by gender, not her state of being a mother. She was defined by her problem using the more pejorative term "drug-addicted" rather than the softer term "substance using." Lastly, she was acknowledged to be pregnant, but not honored as a mother. This exemplifies how words reinforce stereotypes about fitness for motherhood and destroy trust and safety in the healthcare environment.

Media has helped to promote messages of fitness and autonomy in the healthcare environment and in the national conversation. An example is the article by Black journalist Sandy Banks titled *Black Midwives Deliver Comfort and Care in a Kindred Space* (Banks, 2021, Aug 26). This article builds upon themes of fitness, trust, and safety in childbirth. All mothers need a sense of fitness and acceptance. This is even more important if the outcome is not ideal. I have been with mothers whose babies have died. I have heard these words of pain, "I so much wanted to be a mother." My response to them has been, "You *are* a mother and you will always be a mother, even if you have lost your baby." They wear the mantle of motherhood. The media has a powerful role in telling the stories of the strength, autonomy, and fitness of American mothers.

10.4   Summary

Journalism is charged with asking questions: *who, what, when, where, and how much.* Sometimes they even answer the question *why* or at least they allude to it. In the case of journalism depicting maternal health and the factors that undermine it, the American cultural value of individualism is a frequent theme. Storytelling is often used, a powerful tool for relating the questions and helping the public to sort through accurate information, misinformation, and disinformation. The journalist's skill in telling these stories is critical in an open society, especially in the currently polarized environment. Journalists frequently hold the public trust and they are essential in reporting and shaping the national conversation.

Box 10.2 The Power of Journalism

When a story is told, the responsibility of the journalist is to honor the trust of the storyteller, hear beyond words, listen with intuition, and ask questions with open-heartedness. To do so, we must throw away our map and walk a winding path led by the storyteller. This is the power of journalism, leaning into serendipity along the journey.

Even if accurate, statistics and facts alone never tell the full story. Distortion, through misinformation or deliberate disinformation, further betrays the story. The privilege of journalism is to speak the truth, recounting the story entrusted. To do otherwise is to damage and dishonor both the story and the storyteller.

The conversation on maternal health among American mothers is often shallow and hurried, not fully grasping the significance of the story or even distorting the story, breaking the trust of those brave enough to share. This is journalism without truth, without transparency, without power. It fails to inoculate against cultural conflicts, to shine a light on falsehood, to acknowledge the truth of lived experiences, to heal a divided nation.

The pen of the journalist is mighty, mightier than the sword, and it has the power to speak truth to power.

(Personal communication, Martha Hoffman Goedert, PhD, CNM, May 24, 2022)

References

Abrams, A. (2021, Nov 22). [with reporting from journalists Mariah Espada, Washington, D.C. and Leslie Dickstein, New York]. *On the line: Mississippi's last abortion clinic has faced court battles before, but this time it's different.* Time Magazine, pp. 34–38.

Agency for Healthcare Research Quality. (2012, July 31). Evidence-based practice center systematic review protocol. https://www.effectivehealthcare.ahrq.gov

American College of Obstetricians and Gynecologists, Committee on Health Care for Underserved Women. (2014). *Health disparities in rural women—ACOG Committee Opinion # 586* https://www.acog.org/clinical/clinical-guidance/committee-opinion/articles/2014/02/health-disparities-in-rural-women

Amnesty International. (2011). *Deadly delivery: The maternal health care crisis in the USA: One-year update.* Amnesty International Publications. https://cdn2.sph.harvard.edu/wp-content/uploads/sites/32/2017/06/deadlydeliveryoneyear.pdf

Amnesty International. (2018a). *Toxic Twitter-A toxic place for women.* Amnesty International Publications. https://www.amnesty.org/en/latest/research/2018/03/online-violence-against-women-chapter-1/

Amnesty International. (2018b). *Troll Patrol findings: Using crowdsourcing, data science & machine learning to measure violence and abuse against women in Twitter.* Amnesty International Publications. Retrieved from https://decoders.amnesty.org/projects/troll-patrol/findings

Aquilino, W. S. (1996). The life course of children born to unmarried mothers: Childhood living arrangements and young adult outcomes. *Journal of Marriage and the Family, 58*, 293–310.

Associated Press. (2022a. April 22). Judge temporarily blocks Kentucky abortion ban. LATimes. com, p. A-7.

Associated Press. (2022b, Feb 15). Maryland aims to protect abortion rights. LATimes.com. pp. A-7.

Banks, S. (2021, Aug 26). Black midwives deliver comfort and care in a Kindred Space. LATimes. com. pp. A-1, A-8.

Barrett, D., Ortmann, L., & Larson, S. (Eds.). (2022). *Narrative ethics in public health: The value of stories.* Springer.

Beck, C. T. (2002). Postpartum depression: A meta-synthesis of qualitative research. *Qualitative Health Research, 12*, 453–472. https://doi.org/10.1177/104973202129120016

Bland, D. (2020). Exploring misogyny and women's representation in editorial/political cartoons. In M. Marron (Ed.), *Misogyny and media in the age of Trump* (pp. 283–303). Lexington Books.

Building U.S. Capacity to Review and Prevent Maternal Deaths. (2018). *Report from nine maternal mortality review committees.* http://reviewtoaction.org/Report_from_Nine_MMRCs

Calmes, J. (2021, Aug 13). *#MeToo hasn't changed political culture yet.* LATIMES.com, A-11.

Calo, R., Coward, C., Spiro, E., Starbird, K., & West, J. (2021). How do you solve a problem like misinformation? *Science Advances, 7*, 50. https://www.science.org/doi/10.1126/sciadv.abn0481

Cargle, R. (2022, June 18). *Being child-free is my best life.* LATIMES.com,/opinion, A-11.

Carlson, D. L., Petts, R., & Pepin, J. R. (2021, Sept 26). Changes in parents' domestic labor during the COVID-19 pandemic. *Sociological Inquiry, 92*, 1217. https://doi.org/10.1111/soin.12459

Cassese, E. C., & Barnes, T. D. (2019). Intersectional motherhood: Investigating public support for child care subsidies. *Politics, Groups, and Identities, 7*(4), 775–793.

Cowling, C., Machado, M., Paton, D., & West, E. (2017, May 25). Mothering slaves: Comparative perspectives on motherhood, childlessness, and the care of children in Alantic slave societies. *Slavery & Abolition, 38*, 223–231.

Creanga, A. (2018). Maternal mortality in the United States: A review of contemporary data and their limitations. *Clinical Obstetrics and Gynecology, 61*(2), 296–306. https://doi.org/10.1097/GRF.0000000000000362

Davidson, B. (2017). Storytelling and evidence-based policy: Lessons from the grey literature. *Palgrave Communications, 3:*17093. https://doi.org/10.1057/palcomms.2017.93. open access.

De Tocqueville, A. (2003, orig 1835, 1849). Democracy in America. Translated by Gerald Bevan from French original 1835–1840. : Penguin Classics.

Doyle, N. (2018). *Maternal bodies: Redefining motherhood in early America.* The University of North Carolina Press.

Evans, M. (2021, Nov 2). Breast milk as COVID fighter. LATimes.com. pp A-1, A-12.

Fererici, F. (Ed.). (2022). *Language as a social determinant of health: Translating and interpreting the COVID-19 pandemic.* Palgrave Macmillan. https://doi.org/10.1007/978-3-030-87817-7

Friedman, J.& Hansen, H. (2021, Nov 23).Overdose deaths area racial justice issue. LATimes. com. pp A-11.

Garcetto. G., Reiner, I., & Krinsky, M. (2021, Oct 25). Stop obstructing criminal justice reforms. LATimes.com/Opinion, p. A-11.

Geiger, A. W., Livingston, G., & Bialik, K. (2019). 6 facts about U.S. moms. Numbers, Facts and Trends Shaping Your World. https://www.pewresearch.org/fact-tank/2019/05/08/facts-about-u-s-mothers/

Gross, J. L. (2018). Maternal bodies: Redefining motherhood in early America. *Civil War Book Review, 20*(4), 27.

Gutierrez, K. (2022). *June 20* (p. 30). Time Magazine.

Harper, K. (2020). *The ethos of Black motherhood in America: Only White women get pregnant.* Rowman & Littlefield.

Hays, S. (1996). *The cultural contradictions of motherhood.* Yale University Press.

Healthy People. (2030). U.S. Department of Health and Human Services, Office of Disease Prevention and Health Promotion. https://health.gov/healthypeople/objectives-and-data/social-determinants-health

Herbert, D. (2021, Oct 5). In the shadow of childbirth. LATIMES.com. p. A-11.

King, E. (2021, Nov 12). Abortion bans hit military women hard. LATimes.com. p. A-11.

Klemp, N., & Klemp, K. (2021a). *The 80/80 marriage: A new model for a happier, stronger relationship*. Penguin Books.

Klemp, N. & Klemp, K. (2021b, Nov 11). A 'new normal" for housework. Los Angeles Times. p. A-15 www.LATIMES.com

Kumar, S. (2020). The motherhood penalty: Not so Black and White. Electronic Thesis and Dissertation Repository. 7157. https://ir.lib.uwo.ca/etd/7157

Lauter, D. (2021a, Oct 13). Most polarized country? Los Angeles Times. p. A-2. www.LATIMES.com

Lauter, D. (2021b, Oct 25). Americans increasingly divided on race. Los Angeles Times. p. A-2. www.LATIMES.com

Lazariu, V., Nguyen, T., McNutt, L., Jeffrey, J., & Kacica, M. (2017). Severe maternal morbidity: A population-based study of an expanded measure and associated factors. *PLoS One, 12*(8), e0182343. https://doi.org/10.1371/journal.pone.0182343

Liu, C. H., & Tronick, E. (2014). Prevalence and predictors of maternal postpartum depressed mood and anhedonia by race and ethnicity. *Epidemiology and Psychiatric Sciences, 23*(2), 201–209. https://doi.org/10.1017/S2045796013000413

Lopez, A. (2018). *Female journalists and online Duterte trolls*. The American Association of Editorial Cartoonists. https://editorialcartoonists.com/cartoon/display.cfm/173591/

Los Angeles Times Editorial. (2021, Oct 22). Miscarriage is a tragedy, not a criminal offense. LATimes.com. p. A-10.

MacDorman, M., Declercq, E., Cabral, H., & Morton, C. (2016). Recent increases in the U.S. maternal mortality rate—disentangling trends from measurement issues. *Obstetrics & Gynecology, 128*, 447–455. https://doi.org/10.1097/AOG.0000000000001556

Margolis, M. L. (2000). *True to her nature: Changing advice to American women*. Waveland Press.

Marquez, D., Marquez, K. & Gover, T. (2021, Nov 10). Indigenous women face egregious harm. LATimes.com. p. A-14.

Marron, M. (Ed.). (2020). *Misogyny and media in the age of Trump*. Lexington Books.

Matthiesen, S. (2022, Jan 25). *Abortion is not a "choice" without racial justice*. The Boston Review. https://bostonreview.net/articles/abortion-is-not-a-choice-without-racial-justice/

McAvoy, A. (2021, Oct 9). Hawaii targets crimes against Native women. LATimes.com. p. A-2.

Miller, C. C. (2020, November 17). When schools closed, Americans turned to their usual back up plan: Mothers. *New York Times*. https://www.nytimes.com/2020/11/17/upshot/schools-closing-mothers-leaving-jobs.html

Murali, C., & Venkatesan, S. (2022). *Infertility comics and graphic medicine*. Routledge. https://doi.org/10.4324/9781003028628

Newman, H., & Nelson, K. A. (2021). Mother needs a bigger "helper": A critique of "wine mom" discourse as conformity to hegemonic intensive motherhood. *Sociology Compass, 2021*(15), e12868. https://doi.org/10.1111/soc4.12868

Nowogrodzki, A. (2021, Nov 11). Are mothers too easy to blame? *Nature, 599*, 199–200.

Ordoñez, M., & Serrat, O. (2017). Disseminating knowledge products. In I. N. Olivier Serrat (Ed.), *Knowledge solutions: Tool, methods and approaches to drive organizational performance* (pp. 871–878). Springer. https://doi.org/10.1007/978-981-10-0983-9_97

Packer, D. & Van Bavel, J. (2021, Nov 15). Maybe the pandemic 'freethinkers' are really sheep. LATimes.com. p. A-13.

Pollard, M. S., Tucker, J. S., & Green, H. D. (2020). Changes in adult alcohol use and consequences during the COVID-19 pandemic in the US. *JAMA Network Open, 3*(9), e2022942.

Posetti, J., Aboulez, N., Bontcheva, K., Harrison, J., & Waisbord, S. (2020). *Online violence against women journalists: A global snapshot of incidence and impacts*. United Nations Educational, Scientific, and Cultural Organization. Paris: UNESCO. https://unesdoc.unesco.org/ark:/48223/pf0000375136/PDF/375136eng.pdf.multi open access

Regev, M. (2015, Jan. 15). The myth of motherhood: The way unrealistic social expectations of mothers shape their experience. Dr. Regev. https://drregev.com/blog/the-myth-of-motherhood--the-way-unrealistic-social-expectations-of-mothers-shape-their-experience/

Rodriguez, R. (1990). Imaging ourselves IN. In B. Moyer (Ed.), *A world of ideas II: Public opinions from private citizens* (p. 85). Doubleday.

Sawhill, I., Thomas, A., & Monea, E. (2010). An ounce of prevention: Policy prescriptions to reduce the prevalence of fragile families. *The Future of Children, 20*, 133–155.

Segall, E. (2012). Supreme myths: Why the Supreme Court is not a court and its justices are not judges. : ABC-CLIO, LLC.

Sharp, S. (2021, Oct 3) Disabled moms face healthcare snubs. LATimes.com. pp. A-1, A-10-11.

Silver, L., Fetterolf, J. & Connaughton, A. (2021, Oct 13). Diversity and division in advanced economies. Pew Research Center. file:///C:/Users/bande/Desktop/Downloads/PG_2021.10.13_Diversity_Final.pdf

Subbaraman, N. (2021, Nov 25). Homicide is a top cause of maternal death in the United States. *Nature, 599*, 539–540.

Sufrin, C. (2017). *Jailcare: Finding the safety net for women behind bars*. University of California Press.

Tanner, L (2022, April 21). Abortion training scarce, and in decline. LATimes.com. p. A-2.

Taussig, R. (2020). *Sitting pretty: The view from my ordinary resilient disabled body*. HarperCollins Publishers.

Taussig, R. (2021, April 28). Baby steps: Learning to parent in public after a year in our cozy cave. Time Magazine. https://time.com/5958537/pandemic-baby-disabled-mom-rebekah-taussig/

Tenety, E. (2021). It's 2021, but for American mothers, it's still the 1950s. The Mother https://www.mother.ly/life/for-american-mothers-its-1950s/

Thomas, R. K. (2021). *Population health and the future of healthcare*. Springer.

Vandenberg-Daves, J. (2014). *Modern motherhood: An American history*. Rutgers University Press.

Vosoughi, S., Roy, D., & Aral, S. (2018, Mar 9). The spread of true and false news online. *Science, 359*(6380), 1146–1151. https://doi.org/10.1126/science.aap9559

Wagster, E. & Willingham, L. (2022, Feb 2) *Minorities bear brunt of limits on abortion*. LA Times.com, p. A-2.

Walker, D., & Boling, K. (2022). Black maternal mortality in the media: How journlaist cover a deadly racial disparity. *Journalism, 0*(0),1–18. doi: https://doi.org/10.1177/146488492110633.

Weber, P., & Associated Press. (2022, Feb 11). Abortions in Texas fell 60% in the first month under restrictive new law. LATimes.com. para 1. https://www.latimes.com/world-nation/story/2022-02-11/abortions-texas-fell-first-month-new-law).

Weeks, F., Zapata, J. Rohan, A. & Green, T. (2022, Feb 10). Are experiences of racial discrimination associated with postpartum depressive symptoms? A multistate analysis of pregnancy risk assessment monitoring system data. *Journal of Women's Health, 31*(2), 158 https://doi.org/10.1089/jwh.2021.0426 open access.

Westervelt, A. (2018). *Forget "having it all": How America messed up motherhood and how to fix it*. Seal Press.

Williams, H. H. (2021). Just mothering: Amy Coney Barrett and the racial politics of American motherhood. *Laws, 10*(2), 36.

Wire S. (2021, Sept 18). *How willing are taxpayers to foot bill for child care?* LATimes.com. A-2.

Zuckerwise, L. C., & Lipkind, H. S. (2017). Maternal early warning systems—Towards reducing preventable maternal mortality and severe maternal morbidity through improved clinical surveillance and responsiveness. *Seminars in Perinatology, 41*(3), 161–165. https://doi.org/10.1053/j.semperi.2017.03.005

Part IV
Community Forces Influencing Maternal Health

Chapter 11
Healthcare Providers: Leadership for Optimal Maternal Health

Joan MacEachen and Barbara A. Anderson

11.1 Influencing Decisions for Safe Maternal Outcomes

On a daily basis, healthcare providers make critical decisions that influence maternal health outcomes. Their voices and decisions are generally held in high regard by the American public. Rigorous education and legal and regulatory statutes governing practice are supported by both the government and the public. The American society expects health providers to embody the American cultural value of action-orientation and grants them broad scope in decision-making.

This public trust in action-oriented decision-making enables healthcare providers to use knowledge and power to implement changes (Kuhl, 1994), sometimes quickly in situations of danger (Koole & Van den Berg, 2005). Concern for maternal health led to swift implementation of public health and direct care strategies in response to a rapidly evolving environment during the COVID-19 pandemic. Telehealth, limiting contacts in the birth environment, disseminating vaccine information, and countering misinformation are examples of action-oriented decisions to protect mothers. Health education strategies assumed that healthcare providers can employ deliberative messages to influence mothers and that mothers can choose to take deliberative action to protect themselves and their babies. This assumption is grounded in two key social determinants of health (SDoH), accessible healthcare and adequate health literacy, not always available to all mothers. The consequences of these assumptions and the resulting strategic decisions, both positive and negative, are examined in this chapter.

J. MacEachen
Healthcare Provider, Durango, CO, USA

B. A. Anderson (✉)
Frontier Nursing University, Versailles, KY, USA

© The Author(s), under exclusive license to Springer Nature Switzerland AG 2023
B. A. Anderson, L. R. Roberts (eds.), *Maternal Health and American Cultural Values*,
Global Maternal and Child Health, https://doi.org/10.1007/978-3-031-23969-4_11

11.2   Action to Protect Maternal Health During COVID-19

During the initial outbreak of COVID-19 there was heightened concern that pregnant women potentially could suffer severe complications due to the physiologic and immunologic alterations which occur in pregnancy. A previous outbreak of a coronavirus, SARS, was associated with a high incidence of spontaneous miscarriage, preterm delivery, and intrauterine growth restriction (Wong et al., 2004, July). There was also concern that pregnant mothers could be more susceptible to COVID-19 than the general population (Kotlar et al., 2021, Jan 18). As a result of these concerns, the care offered to mothers was altered significantly and frequently to protect both childbearing women and the healthcare workforce. Globally, 70% of the healthcare workforce are women, necessitating further consideration for their safety as well as clients (World Health Organization [WHO], 2019).

Swift changes involved policy and guidelines across the childbearing spectrum. Various organizations such as WHO and the Center for Disease Control and Prevention (CDC) evaluated current information and published recommendations for care providers, hospitals, and clinics which were then responsible for incorporating these guidelines according to their perceived level of threat. In the USA, the implementation of policy and practice guidelines reflected the cultural value of action-orientation. An exemplar is the comprehensive evidence-based review in publication and smartphone app, *UpToDate*, which outlined the issues and recommendations for providers (Berghella & Hughes, 2022, July).

11.2.1   *Provision of Maternal HealthCare Access during COVID-19*

Tracking revealed that morbidity, mortality, and intensive care admissions were highest among mothers who were non-White in ethnicity, had chronic hypertension, pre-existing diabetes and/or high body mass index, and advanced maternal age (Muralidar et al., 2020, Sept 22). A simultaneous cross-sectional study revealed that 54.5% of pregnant women who tested positive for COVID-19 on admission were asymptomatic (Delahoy, et al., 2020, Sept 25). Using an action-oriented approach, the healthcare system instituted a triage system to alter protocols to limit the spread of COVID-19. The policies included:

- Reducing the number of face-to-face visits.
- Grouping laboratory tests for less client contact.
- Revising timing and decreasing frequency of ultrasounds and nonstress tests.
- Restricting support persons in hospital and clinic facilities.
- Employing virtual and telemedicine consultations and visits.

These were guidelines that health providers for the most part supported, utilizing the referent power of their professional status to actively enforce the changes. The full effect of these practice changes on maternal health outcomes has yet to be evaluated. However, one of the unintended but evident consequences of limiting the number of pre-postnatal visits and the presence of support persons was increased maternal anxiety. Prior to the pandemic, antenatal depression already affected 10% of women in the developed world, and the number of women taking antidepressants had been increasing over the previous ten years (Noordam et al., 2015, Jan 6). This is important because prenatal depression is linked to a greater risk of postnatal depression and loss of interest in the child (DaCosta et al., 2000). During the pandemic, studies revealed moderate to severe anxiety related to the potential of infecting the fetus, limited accessibility and cancellation of appointments, restrictions on support persons attending appointment, and social distancing and quarantine guidelines during birth (Groulx et al., 2021; Kotlar et al., 2021 Jan 18; Saccone et al., 2020). Another study subsequently showed a decrease in maternal anxiety once the COVID-19 numbers had peaked, assumed to be due to social media and healthcare providers in actively providing accurate information (Kotabagi et al., 2020, July).

Telehealth visits were implemented prior to the pandemic. Pandemic guidelines recommended expanded use of telehealth or video for pre- and postnatal care which did not necessitate a physical exam, lab work, or imaging. Virtual media was used for online childbirth classes and tours of birthing units. Expanded use of telephone or video helplines and provider availability for answering email from clients about psychosocial concerns and COVID-19 were action-oriented strategies encouraged by the healthcare system (UpToDate, 2022). Randomized controlled studies demonstrated the efficacy of telehealth encounters in breastfeeding support, smoking cessation, continuation of oral and injectable contraception, provision of medical abortion, and monitoring of high-risk pregnancies in reducing preeclampsia among mothers with gestational hypertension (DeNicola et al., 2020, Feb 1). A survey of 1060 maternal and newborn healthcare providers on their assessment of increased telehealth communication showed that while 58% of the informants had used telehealth, only 60% of those who had used this strategy had received any training. The challenges of telehealth include lack of infrastructure and technical proficiency, limited access to client monitoring, client health literacy, financial and language barriers to technology, establishing trust in the provider-patient relationship, and the lack of non-verbal feedback (Galle et al., 2021, Feb). However, another study by nurse-anthropologist Jennifer Foster revealed that telehealth among low-income pregnant and parenting adolescents revealed that most of these young mothers had cell phones and were very receptive to telehealth (Foster et al., 2015).

11.2.2 Management of Vaccine Hesitancy and Misinformation

The pharmaceutical companies quickly went into action to develop vaccinations against COVID-19. Childbearing women were largely excluded from the initial clinical trials due to safety and ethical concerns (Gardner, 2021, Nov 1). Once the vaccinations were shown to be safe and effective for large segments of the global population, the education of the public and civic participation advocating maternal vaccination became key action-oriented strategies by healthcare providers across the world (Jacob et al., 2020, Sept 21). Unvaccinated women planning to become pregnant and childbearing women were encouraged to get initial vaccination and booster doses when eligible (American College of Obstetricians and Gynecologists, 2020, Dec, updated 2022, June).

In spite of health information efforts on the part of healthcare providers, much of the information dissemination revolved around correcting the accuracy of information and quelling reports of misinformation and disinformation in media sources. On July 15, 2021, Dr. Vivek Murthy, Surgeon General, from the Office of the Surgeon General, issued a press release warning the public about the risk of misinformation and disinformation (see https://www.hhs.gov/about/news/2021/07/15/us-surgeon-general-issues-advisory-during-covid-19-vaccination-push-warning-american.html). In alignment with the WHO campaign, *Stop the Spread* (see https://www.who.int/news-room feature-stories/detail/countering-misinformation-about-covid-19) and the United States Health and Human Services campaign, *We Can Do This* (see https://wecandothis.hhs.gov), the Surgeon General also issued a comprehensive public document advising multiple stakeholders on action-oriented approaches to decrease misinformation and disinformation about COVID-19. In particular, he recommended that healthcare providers, public health professionals, and health organizations seek to build public trust using appropriate health literacy levels and engage in civic life through technology, media, and community organizations (Murthy, 2021). He stated, "If you are a clinician, take the time to understand each patient's knowledge, beliefs, and values. Listen with empathy, and when possible, correct misinformation in personalized ways. When addressing health concerns, consider using less technical language that is accessible to all patients" (Murthy, 2021, p. 10). The CDC Division of Reproductive Health backed-up this outreach with the *Hear Her Campaign*. It identifies specific strategies for helping healthcare providers with active listening skills, recognition of adverse SDoH, awareness of potential bias and inequity in client-provider relationships, and key messages to deliver to pregnant and postpartum women on urgent maternal warning signs (see https://www.cdc/hearher/healthcare-providers/index.html).

Despite strong recommendation by healthcare providers, vaccination for COVID-19 uptake among pregnant women has been low (Razzaghi et al., 2021, June 18). Vaccine hesitancy has a history in the USA. Ben Franklin hesitated to allow his son to have smallpox inoculation and his son later died of the disease. Franklin subsequently became an advocate for inoculation within a skeptical community (Best et al., 2007). Even today, many mothers do not trust the safety of vaccines, especially new vaccines. Elena Conis, an American historian of medicine and public health, in her review of the history of vaccine hesitancy in the USA, included the now debunked controversy over an autism link, the influence of parents and dissented healthcare providers who questioned vaccine safety, and the legitimacy of governmental jurisdiction and enforcement (Conis, 2015a, b). Healthcare providers have struggled with the public hesitancy and the emotional persistence of belief in misinformation while attempting to be action-oriented in providing steady guidance

(Chou & Budenz, 2020; Gardner, 2021, Nov 1; Southwell et al., 2020). As described by Manoncourt et al. (2022), critical action-orientation approaches by healthcare providers in addressing hesitancy are visibility and leadership in social mobilization and community organization, recognition of SDoH and cultural barriers, and fostering trust through respectful interactions.

11.3   Action to Protect Mothers at Especially High Risk

Proactive counseling and intervention to prevent adverse outcomes are an integral part of guarding maternal care. Healthcare providers are grounded in the American social expectation to assume these responsibilities. More than many other professions, they are held accountable to reflect the American cultural value of action-orientation. In exchange, they are granted broad scope in decision-making in providing maternal healthcare.

11.3.1   Guarding Mothers at High Risk

Childbearing is a normal physiologic process, not a disease. The role of the healthcare provider is to support progress toward a healthy outcome, enhance family development, and observe for and intervene with pathology. Most pregnancies follow the curve of normal, but when they do not, dire consequences can emerge, sometimes with great alacrity. One starry-eyed young student interviewed me (BA) about my work as a healthcare provider. She said she wanted to care for mothers because it was so "happy" and she wanted to feel happy in her work. In all honesty, I had to weave into the interview some stories of when it was not so happy. Hopefully, I left her with the impression that the care of mothers is both the agony and the ecstasy of life—that my job was to be a trusted and competent health guardian, no matter what the outcome.

Perhaps the most difficult part of guarding the health of mothers at high risk is addressing unhealthy lifestyle patterns and adverse SDoH. As discussed throughout this work, most maternal morbidity and mortality is preventable and much of maternal healthcare in the USA is consumed in supporting mothers at especially high risk, most of whom struggle with health disruptions due to lifestyle and SDoH. Healthcare providers are reasonably well prepared to address unhealthy lifestyle patterns and, as discussed above, there are excellent materials to enhance skills. Supporting empowerment, self-determination, goal setting, reflexive thought, social support, and shared decision-making have been shown to be more effective than merely giving facts (Castro et al., 2016; Zinsser et al., 2020). As a young professional, I (BA) remember feeling so discouraged after carefully imparting facts about her risks to a 45-year-old obese, hypertensive prenatal client. She patently ignored everything I said. When she experienced an eclamptic seizure, barely surviving, I shared my feeling of failure with my supervisor. I lamented, "But I told her. I gave her all the facts." My supervisor wisely said words that I have never forgotten: "Information does not change behavior." Fortunately, the strategies identified above, based upon extensive research on health behavior change, have improved the ability and skills of healthcare providers.

Screening for prenatal substance use is an example of an action-oriented strategy to address unhealthy lifestyle and adverse SDoH issues (Haycraft, 2018; Krans & Patrick, 2018). Providers are often hesitant to screen for substance abuse, fearing confrontation with the mother. It is a culturally stigmatized behavior that society places outside of the standards for being a "good mother" (Nichols et al., 2021). Stigmatization of substance using mothers, a violation of key American cultural values and maternal role definitions, is addressed in depth in Chaps. 3, 14, and 15. Yet, in a recent survey, nearly all pregnant women found screening acceptable for alcohol (97%), tobacco (98%), and other drug use (97%) during prenatal care (Toquinto et al., 2020). As a healthcare provider, I (JME) am still tempted to address the admission of substance use in mothers by advice for what I feel must be an information deficit. After realizing the futility of this approach, I now initiate any intervention with the question, "How can I help you?" Accepting her response is the key to further evaluation and treatment.

11.3.2   Exemplar: American Indian/Alaskan Native Mothers at Risk

Although there are many groups of childbearing women at especially high risk, for the purpose of this chapter, one exemplar of action-orientation is presented. Compared to other childbearing women, American Indian/Alaskan Native (AI/AN) mothers have high rates of intimate partner violence (IPV), rape, history of adverse childhood events (ACE), substance abuse, and post-partum depression (Evans-Campbell et al., 2006; Maxwell & Leat, 2022, Mar 6). AI/AN mothers have often experienced the effects of intergenerational trauma, lack of role models for mothering, a sense of abandonment, and post-traumatic stress disorder (PTSD) (Henry et al., 2021). All of these factors increase the risk of alcohol abuse, tobacco use, suicide, and homicide (Evans-Campbell et al., 2006; Gone & Trimble, 2012; Henry et al., 2021; James et al., 2021, Oct 21). Substance abusing mothers in general endure stigma about fitness for motherhood, but the rates of intervention by child welfare services, and increased rates of incarceration, are higher among Black and AI/AN mothers (Terplan et al., 2015, Sept 20). While substance using mothers in general endure stigma about fitness for motherhood, intervention by child welfare services, and increased rates of incarceration, the rates are higher among Black and AI/AN mothers (Terplan et al., 2015, Sept 20).

Substance abuse is a way of coping and managing emotional and physical pain (Henry et al., 2021). Mothers who use substances come into the healthcare system wounded, often facing hurdles in accessing treatment programs. Stigma and rejection further inflict pain. Healthcare providers can be highly influential in using action-oriented decision-making power that can help or revictimize. That is why the question "How can I help you?" may be a life line. Listening through the lens of the SDoH can help, even in the face of scarce resources (Haycraft, 2018; Krans & Patrick, 2016). As a family medicine doctor and public health specialist, I (JME) have worked with various AI/AN tribes for 28 years. I have come to appreciate the role of the healthcare provider in offering an action-oriented but culturally relevant approach that incorporates trauma-informed treatment. Such treatment recognizes that many substance abusing mothers may know about but not utilize healthy coping methods and often deeply desire to be good mothers. Being emotionally available and engendering trust brings authenticity to the question "How can I help you?"

Offering appropriate referrals is another powerful action-oriented strategy amendable to healthcare providers. Understanding the influence of the SDoH domains, *Neighborhood* and *Community*, as described in the *Healthy People 2030* document (Healthy People, 2030), brings balance into collaboration with often-conflictual Child Protective Services (CPS) and community services. There is limited research on the efficacy of substance abuse treatment among AI/AN mothers, especially inpatient services. One factor that is often overlooked is the power of the SDoH, *Neighborhood* and *Community*. In the case of AI/AN, the collectivism of the community and interdependence in the family network may influence individual client decision-making, as well-described by Hossain et al. (2011) in research on Navajo families. The close-knit relationships on a reservation can make it difficult to maintain distance from the sources of trauma and substances. Mothers have expressed to me (JME) that *when sober* they feel isolated, unsupported in sobriety, and guilt over abandoning family members who continue to use.

These AI/AN also worry about the safety of their children if they enter an inpatient treatment center. I (BA) had to accept the refusal of a highly addicted American Indian mother for inpatient substance abuse treatment. She explained her fear that her children would be raped by relatives so she could not leave them. No facilities would take her with her young children. She eventually lost custody and her children remained in the custody of relatives, among whom were previously convicted child rapists. A study of Alaska Native patients admitted to inpatient alcohol detoxification identified that mothers were especially in need of inpatient services that admitted the clients with their children and provided services for IPV (Running-Bear et al., 2016).

One substance abuse treatment program for AI/AN stands out in addressing the interaction of SDoH, social stigma of substance using mothers, and the cultural value of action-orientation in the healthcare system (Schultz et al., 2018, Oct 18). In an effort to develop a treatment program, a Washington State American Indian tribe commissioned research on risk and protective factors related to substance abuse among mothers in their community. They secured funding from three sources: the National Institutes on Drug Abuse, Mental Health, and Minority Health and Health Disparities and collaborated with social worker researchers. Using community-based participatory research, 20 in-depth interviews and one focus group among AI/

AN women of childbearing age who lived on or near a reservation in the Pacific Northwest were conducted. Of the sample, 15/20 were mothers and the others were young, preconceptual women. In addition, in-depth interviews were conducted with a small sample of tribal elders for cultural context. A community advisory board was established with the tribal population and the University of Washington. Community-wide action-orientation by all of the stakeholders in this study was a key strength (Schultz et al., 2018, Oct 18). This study identified four driving themes among these American Indian women that pointed toward an enlightening conclusion:

- A tight relationship between the lived experience of trauma and substance use.
- The value of traditional healing as pathway to recovery.
- Community-based and cultural patterns as challenges to recovery.
- Motherhood as a motivating factor in seeking treatment and sustaining recovery (Schultz et al., 2018, Oct 18).

Pregnancy and motherhood were key factors in both precipitating substance use but also in motivation for seeking treatment and succeeding in recovery. The support of traditional healing rituals buffers in prevention of substance abuse and supporting recovery. The informants cited cultural traditions such as pow wows, communal sweat rituals, and the Pacific NorthWest tradition of canoe journeys were specific examples of ways to reach spiritual connections and connect their children with elders and mentors in the community. They reflected upon the difficulty of maintaining distance from the sources of trauma and substances within the community but also on how embracing the role of motherhood is a motivating factor in seeking treatment and retaining sobriety. They reported that the loss of children to CPS and the subsequent neglect or abuse of the children was the strongest motivation to seek and persist with treatment (Schultz et al., 2018, Oct 18). As a dichotomy, AI/AN families, who are over-represented in and often have adversarial relationships with CPS, have reported that it may be a pathway to access treatment and a motivator to maintain sobriety. Embracing the mantle of motherhood may be the key to healthy outcomes for these women (Schultz et al., 2018, Oct 18). The implication for healthcare providers is that the cultural value of action-orientation in supporting AI/AN mothers includes collaboration and deep respect for their cultural values.

11.4   Action to Support Conditions for Optimal Birth

11.4.1   Public Advocacy for Healthcare System Action

Choices for place of birth and birthing practices have a long history of healthcare provider inaction in the USA. Many of the current practices, such as free-standing and hospital-attached birth centers, doulas, awake-and-aware birth, and woman-to-woman support for breastfeeding arose, not out of health provider action, but out of public advocacy. The books *Thank you Dr. Lamaze, The Womanly Art of Breastfeeding* from La Leche League International, and Ina May Gaskin's book, *Spiritual Midwifery*, were best sellers. They discussed the discontent around hospital birthing practices and offered alternatives (Gaskin, 2002. Karmel & Karmel, 1960, Wiessinger et al., 2010). A grassroots consumer movement was sparked and a plethora of popular literature on childbirth followed. Gaskin became an iconic figure promoting out-of-hospital birth at her rural facility *The Farm*, in Tennessee and also for developing the famous Gaskin maneuver for management of the birth complication, shoulder dystocia. This maneuver has been validated to decrease injury to the newborn (Zheng et al., 2021).

There were calls from many sectors challenging the American healthcare system to address health inequity, racism, accurate tracking of maternal mortality, and evidence-based birthing practices supported by systematic reviews (Bohren et al., 2017; Building U.S. Capacity to Review and Prevent Maternal Deaths, 2018; Wallace et al., 2016; Williams, 2016). The birth center movement, as a way returning childbirth to the community, was led by midwifery and the American Association of Birth Centers (Stone et al., 2017; American Association of Birth Centers, 2015). The long tradition of "granny midwives" among the Black population dates back to the 1600s. It enabled survival among enslaved Black mothers and post-emancipation Black mothers who were excluded from healthcare facilities serving only White mothers (Bovard & Milton, 1993; Luke, 2018; Varney & Thompson, 2015). The story of these "Grand" midwives (as they are renamed) has been acknowledged and featured in the Smithsonian Institute (Pretzer, n.d.; Varney & Thompson, 2015). The Black Mamas Matter Alliance (BMMA), a vocal advocacy group, has promoted traditional Black practices as a pathway to physiologic birth and emotional safety (see https://blackmamasmatter.org/).

11.4.2   The Healthcare System Response

Across the globe, healthcare providers and public health professionals began to closely examine not only maternal morbidity and mortality, but also practices surrounding birth—technology, physiologic birth, and emotional safety during birth (Afulani & Moyer, 2019; Bohren et al., 2019; Edmonds et al., 2020; et al., 2014; MacDorman & Declercq, 2016; National Institute for Health and Care Excellence, 2014 updated 2019, Feb 27; Poškienė et al., 2021). Respectful maternity care, obstetrical violence, and human rights were topics in the spotlight (United Nations, 2019, July 11). The American healthcare system was slow to respond to the cascade of public opinion to take action to improve conditions of birth and address public concerns, but gradually healthcare providers began to evaluate the practices of the past. Leadership and action to address systemic problems have now occurred on many fronts, including awareness of health inequity and racism, management of catastrophic maternal events, addressing provider shortage, fatigue and sleep deficits, and data management on maternal health outcomes (Auerbach et al., 2017; Brantley et al., 2017; Kozhimannil et al., 2016; Menard et al., 2015; Nove et al., 2021). Healthcare providers have displayed exemplary leadership and action-orientation in protecting maternal health during the COVID-19 pandemic.

A persistent problem is the geographical maldistribution of the healthcare workforce and maternal healthcare services particularly in Southern and Western regions and rural communities across the nation (Auerbach et al., 2017; Brantley et al., 2017; Kozhimannil et al., 2016). According to the Pew Charitable Trusts, between 50 and 56% of counties in the USA, mostly in rural areas, do not have a healthcare provider to attend births (Ollove, 2016, August 15). Mothers in rural areas often have to travel hours for prenatal and birth care, contributing to rising adverse maternal health outcomes (DiPietro-Mager et al., 2021; et al., 2022). Healthcare provider shortages are severe for up to 500,000 rural women giving birth each year (Kozhimannil et al., 2016) and for the past 20 years, maternity care services in rural hospitals have been closing (Hung et al., 2016). Both community advocates and many healthcare providers have proposed planned home birth and community-based birth centers as viable solutions to these "maternity care deserts." Although usually in rural areas, maternity care deserts also occur in high-density urban areas, often populated by mothers of color who desire more cultural and racial congruity with their healthcare providers. The following interview is an example of action-orientation by a healthcare provider addressing these needs.

Box 11.1 Interview with Nikia Grayson, DNP, CNM, Director of Clinical Services, CHOICES Memphis Center for Reproductive Health, Memphis, TN by Suzan Ulrich, DrPH, CNM, Director of Midwifery Education, George Washington University

Community birth centers are developing in Black communities to meet the challenge of disproportionally high rates of mortality for Black mothers and babies by actively addressing the social determinants of health. Dr. Nikia Grayson is addressing these disparities as the Director of Clinical Services at CHOICES Memphis Center for Reproductive Health. Located in Midtown in Memphis, Tennessee, CHOICES is an independent, nonprofit community health clinic and birth center with a focus on reproductive and sexual health justice. (See https://memphischoices.org/).

Dr. Grayson wears many hats! She is an anthropologist, journalist, certified nurse-midwife, family nurse practitioner and community activist. As an anthropologist, she conducted research for the *March of Dimes* interviewing families about their care and found inequities and high rates of infant mortality among Black families who described how the social determinants of health have influenced their life trajectory and health. These families said that these root causes of health issues were not addressed because no one listened and healthcare providers did not value their experiences. Dr. Nikia stresses that communities know what they need and that the best way to develop healthcare that culturally fits is by talking to the people in the community.

Dr. Grayson decided to take action. She became a nurse-midwife to assure that her community had a culturally congruent midwife who would meet their needs with respectful care. In 2017, she started the midwifery component at CHOICES initially offering home birth services. She then received hospital privileges so she could care for women both in the community and in the hospital. In 2020, two more nurse midwives joined her and in February 2021 a community-based birth center was opened at CHOICES. The center strives to actively address social determinants of health. Experiencing this personalized and respectful care has inspired some of these mothers to take action themselves by studying to become lactation consultants, doulas, nurses, midwives, and physicians.

This same grass roots action-orientated approach is happening across the nation as community-based birth centers, often established by midwives of color, seek to provide high quality, culturally congruent care that improves maternal health outcomes and builds strong families and communities. Research by the Strong Start Birth Centers Initiative, conducted by the Centers for Medicare and Medicaid Innovation (CMMI), found that the birth center model of care decreased rates of prematurity, low birth weight, and racial disparities (Hill et al., 2018). Care in birth centers strives to provide holistic, patient centered with shared decision-making, cultural sensitivity and promotion of normal physiologic birth and breastfeeding. This approach to care is beneficial for Black mothers who have deep distrust of the medical establishment from centuries of abuse, discrimination, and structural racism. It is a positive action-oriented approach to a broken maternity care system by Dr. Grayson and the team at CHOICES.

(Personal communication, Nikia Grayson by Suzan Ulrich, DrPH, CNM, Director of Midwifery Education, George Washington University, October 6, 2021).

11.5 Summary

Each mother brings a unique life story to childbearing. On a daily basis, healthcare providers are witness to adverse SDoH. It is not unusual for the tapestry of the mother's life story to include poverty, limited education and health literacy, racism, ACEs, mental illness, substance abuse, and intimate partner violence. These SDoH erode her health.

Action-orientation is a key American cultural value that validates health promotion with healthcare providers' broad scope in decision-making. The American public expects them to model this cultural value and grants them broad scope in decision-making. Proactive approaches by healthcare providers can be decisive in how a woman adapts to motherhood, her experience in giving birth, whether she thrives, or even whether she survives.

References

Afulani, P., & Moyer, C. (2019). Accountability for respectful maternity care. *The Lancet, 394*(10210), 1692–1693. https://doi.org/10.1016/S0140-6736(19)322

American Association of Birth Centers. (2015). A historical timeline: Highlights of 4 decades of developing the birth center concept in the U.S. American Association of Birth Centers. https://www.Birthcenters.org/general/custom.asp?page=history

American College of Obstetricians and Gynecologists. (2020, Dec, updated June 3, 2022). COVID-19 vaccination considerations for obstetric-gynecologic care. *ACOG Clinical Practice Advisory.* https://www.acog.org/clinical/clinical-guidance/practice-advisoryarticles/2020/12/covid-19-vaccination-considerations-for-obstetric-gynecologic-care

Auerbach, D., Buerhaus, P., & Staiger, D. (2017). How fast will the registered nurse workforce grow through 2030? Projections in nine regions of the country. *Nursing Outlook, 65*, 116–122. https://doi.org/10.1016/j.outlook.2016.07.004

Berghella, V., & Hughes, B. (2022, July). COVID-19: Overview of pregnancy issues. *UpToDate,* https://www.uptodate.com/contents/covid-19-overview-of-pregnancy-issues#H2125805726

Best, M., Katamba, A., & Neuhauser, D. (2007, Dec). Making the right decision: Benjamin Franklin's son dies of smallpox in 1736. *Quality and Safety in Health Care, 16*(6), 478–480. https://doi.org/10.1136/qshc.2007.023465

Bohren, M., Hofmeyr, G., Sakala, C., Fukuzawa, R., & Cuthbert, A. (2017, July 6). Continuous support for women during childbirth. *Cochrane Database of Systematic Reviews, 7*(7), CD003766. https://doi.org/10.1002/14651858.CD003766.pub6

Bohren, M., Mehrtash, H., Fawole, B., Maung, T., Balde, M., Maya, E., Thwin, S., Aderoba, A. K., Vogel, J., & Irinyenikan, T. (2019). How women are treated during facility-based childbirth in four countries: A cross-sectional study with labour observations and community-based surveys. *The Lancet, 394*(10210), 1750–1763.

Bovard, W., & Milton, G. (1993). *Why not me?: The story of Gladys Milton, midwife.* Book Publishing Company.

Brantley, M., Davis, N., Goodman, D., Callaghan, W., & Barfield, W. (2017). Perinatal regionalization: A geospatial view of perinatal critical care, United States, 2010-2013. *American Journal of Obstetrics and Gynecology, 216*(185), e1. https://doi.org/10.1016/j.ajog.2016.10.011

Building U.S. Capacity to Review and Prevent Maternal Deaths. (2018). *Report from nine maternal mortality review committees.* http://reviewtoaction.org/Report_from_Nine_MMRCs

Castro, E., Regenmortel, T., Vanhaecht, K., Sermeus, W., & Hecke, A. (2016). Patient empowerment, patient participation and patient-centeredness in hospital care: A concept analysis based on a literature review. *Patient Education and Counseling, 99*(12), 1923–1939. https://doi.org/10.1016/j.pec.2016.07.026

Chou, W., & Budenz, A. (2020). Considering emotion in COVID-19 vaccine communication: Addressing vaccine hesitancy and fostering vaccine confidence. *Health Communication, 35*(14), 1718–1722. https://doi.org/10.1080/10410236.2020.1838096

Conis, E. (2015a). *Vaccine nation: America's changing relationship with immunization.* The University of Chicago Press.

Conis E. (2015b). Vaccine resistance in historical perspective. *The American Historian.* https://www.oah.org/tah/issues/2015/august/vaccination-resistance/

DaCosta, D., Larouche, J., Dritsa, M., & Brender, W. (2000). Psychosocial correlates of prepartum and postpartum depressed mood. *Journal of Affective Disorders, 59*(1), 31–40. https://doi.org/10.1016/s0165-0327(99)00128-7

Delahoy, M.,Whitaker, M., O'Halloran, A., Chai, S., Kirley, P., Alden, N., COVID-NET Surveillance Team. (2020). Characteristics and maternal and birth outcomes of hospitalized pregnant women with laboratory-confirmed COVID-19 — COVID-NET, 13 States, March 1–August 22, 2020. *Morbidity and Mortality Weekly Report, 69*(38), 1347–1354. https:www.cdc.gov/mmwr/69/wr/pdfs/mm6938e 1-H.pdf

DeNicola, N., Grossman, D., Marko, K., Sonalkar, S., Butler-Tobah, Y., Ganju, N., & Lowery, C. (2020, Feb 1). Telehealth interventions to improve obstetric and gynecologic health outcomes. *Obstetrics and Gynecology, 135*(3), 371–382. https://doi.org/10.1097/AOG.0000000000003646

DiPietro-Mager, N., Zollinger, T., Turman, J., Zhang, J., & Dixon, B. (2021). Routine healthcare utilization among reproductive-age women residing in a rural maternity care desert. *Journal of Community Health, 46*(1), 108–116. https://doi.org/10.1007/s10900-020-00852-6

Edmonds, J. K., Ivanof, J., & Kafulafula, U. (2020). Midwife led units: Transforming maternity care globally. *Annals of Global Health, 86*(1), 44. https://doi.org/10.5334/aogh.2794

Evans-Campbell, T., Lindhorst, T., Huang, B., & Walters, K. L. (2006). Interpersonal violence in the lives of urban American Indian and Alaska native women: Implications for health, mental health, and help-seeking. *American Journal of Public Health, 96*(8), 1416–1422.

Foster, J., Miller, L., Isbell, S., Shields, T., Worthy, N., & Dunlop, A. (2015). mHealth to promote pregnancy and interconception health among African-American women at risk for adverse birth outcomes: A pilot study. *mHealth, 1*, 20. https://doi.org/10.3978/j.issn.2306-9740.2015.12.01

Galle, A., Semaan, A., Huysmans, E., Audet, C., Asefa, A., Delvaux, T., & Benova, L. (2021, Feb). A double-edged sword- telemedicine for maternal care during COVID-19: Findings from a global mixed-methods study of healthcare providers. *BMJ Global Health, 6*(2), e004575. https://doi.org/10.1136/bmjgh-2020-004575

Gardner, L. (2021, Nov 1). Pregnant people were shut out of Covid vaccine trials-- with disastrous results. *Politico, 4*. https://www.politico.com/news/2021/11/01/covid-vaccine-studies-pregnant-people-518215

Gaskin, I. (2002). *Spiritual midwifery*. Book Publishing Company.

Gone, J., & Trimble, J. (2012). American Indian and Alaska native mental health: Diverse perspectives on enduring disparities. *Annual Review of Clinical Psychology, 8*, 131–160.

Groulx, T., Bagshawe, M., Giesbrecht, G., Tomfohr-Madsen, L., Hetherington, E., & Lebel, C. (2021, April 23). Prenatal care disruptions and associations with maternal mental health during the COVID-19 pandemic. *Frontiers in Global Women's Health, 2*, PMC859398. https://doi.org/10.3389/fgwh.2021.648428

Haycraft, A. (2018). Pregnancy and the opioid epidemic. *Journal of Psychosocial Nursing and Mental Health Services, 56*(3), 19–23. https://doi.org/10.3928/02793695-20180219-03

Healthy People. (2030). U.S. Department of Health and Human Services, Office of Disease Prevention and Health Promotion. https://health.gov/healthypeople/objectives-and-data/social-determinants-health

Henry, M., Sanjuan, P., Stone, L., Cairo, G., Lohr-Valdez, A., & Leeman, L. (2021). Alcohol and other substance use disorder recovery during pregnancy among patients with posttraumatic stress disorder symptoms: A qualitative study. *Drug and Alcohol Dependence Reports, 1*, 100013.

Hill, I., Dubay, L., Courtot, B., Benatar, S., Garrett, B., Blavin, F., Howell, E., Johnston, E., Allen, E., Thornburgh, S., Markell, J., Morgan, J., Silow-Carroll, S., Bitterman, J., Rodin, J., Odendahl, R., Paez, K., Thompson, L., et al. (2018). *Strong start for mothers and newborns evaluation: Year 5 project synthesis, volume 1: Cross-cutting findings*. Baltimore (MD). https://downloads.cms.gov/files/cmmi/strongstart-prenatal-finalevalrpt-v1.pdf

Hossain, Z., Skurky, T., Joe, J., & Hunt, T. (2011). The sense of collectivism and individualism among husbands and wives in traditional and bi-cultural Navajo families on the Navajo reservation. *Journal of Comparative Family Studies, 42*(4), 543–562.

Hung, P., Kozhimannil, K., Casey, M., & Moscovice, I. (2016). Why are obstetric units in rural hospitals closing their doors? *Health Services Research, 51*(4), 1546–1560. https://doi.org/10.1111/1475-6773.12441

Jacob, C., Briana, D., Di Renzo, G., Modi, N., Bustreo, F., Conti, G., & Hanson, M. (2020, Sept 21). Building resilient societies after COVID-19: The case for investing in maternal, neonatal, and child health. *The Lancet Public Health, 5*, e624–e627. https://doi.org/10.1016/S2468-2667(20)30200-0

James, R., Hesketh, M., Benally, T., Johnson, S., Tanner, L., & Means, S. (2021). Assessing social determinants of health in a prenatal and perinatal cultural intervention for American Indians and Alaska Natives. *International Journal of Environmental Research in Public Health, 18* (21), 11079. https://doi.org/10.3390/ijerph182111079. PMID: 34769596.

Karmel, M., & Karmel, A. (1960). *Thank you Dr. Lamaze.* Doubleday.

Koole, S., & Van den Berg, A. (2005). Lost in the wilderness: Terror management, action orientation, and nature evaluation. *Journal of Personality and Social Psychology, 88*(6), 1014–1028.

Kotabagi, P., Fortune, L., Essien, S., Nauta, M., & Yoong, W. (2020, July). Anxiety and depression levels among pregnant women with COVID-19. *Acta Obstetricia et Gynecologica Scandinavica, 99*(7), 953–954. https://doi.org/10.1111/aogs.13928

Kotlar, B., Gerson, E., Petrillo, S., Langer, A., & Tiemeier, H. (2021. Jan 18). The impact of the COVID-19 pandemic on maternal and perinatal health: A scoping review. *Reproductive Health, 18*, 10. https://doi.org/10.1186/s12978-021-01070-6

Kozhimannil, K., Henning-Smith, C., Hung, P., Casey, M., & Prasad, S. (2016). Ensuring access to high-quality maternity care in rural America. *Women's Health Issues, 26*(3), 247–250. https://doi.org/10.1016/j.whi.2016.02.001

Krans, E., & Patrick, S. (2016). Opioid use disorder in pregnancy, health policy and practice in the midst of an epidemic. *Obstetrics and Gynecology, 128*(1), 4–10. https://doi.org/10.1097/AOG.0000000000001446

Kuhl, J. (1994). A theory of self-regulation: Action versus state orientation, self-discrimination, and some applications. *Applied Psychology, 41*(2), 97–129.

Luke, J. (2018). *Delivered by midwives: African-American midwifery in the twentieth-century south.* University Press of Mississippi.

MacDorman, M., & Declercq, E. (2016). Trends and characteristics of United States out-of-hospital birth 2004-2014: New information on risk status and access to care. *Birth: Issues in Perinatal Care, 43*(2), 116–124. https://doi.org/10.1111/birt.12228

Manoncourt, E., Obregon, R., & Chitnis, K. (2022). *Communication and community engagement in disease outbreaks: Dealing with rights, culture, complexity, and context.* Springer.

Maxwell, D., & Leat, S. (2022, Mar 6). A review of the empirical measures on becoming a mother and their relevance to the American Indian/native mother: Implications for research and policy. *Journal of Ethnic & Cultural Diversity in Social Work., 31*(2), 63–83. https://doi.org/10.1080/15313204.2022.2041520

Menard, K., Kilpatrick, S., Saade, G., Hollier, L., Joseph, G., Barfield, W., & Conry, J. (2015). Levels of maternal care. *American Journal of Obstetrics and Gynecology, 212*(3), 259–271. https://doi.org/10.1016/j.ajog.2014.12.030

Muralidar, S., Ambi, S., Sekaran, S., & Krishnan, U. (2020, Sept 22). The emergence of COVID-19 as a global pandemic: Understanding the epidemiology, immune response and potential therapeutic targets of SARS-CoV-2. *Biochimie, 179*, 85–100. https://doi.org/10.1016/j.biochi.2020.09.018

Murthy, V. (2021). *Confronting health misinformation: The U.S. surgeon General's advisory on building a healthy information environment.* United States Health and Human Services, Public Health Service. pp. 1-22. https://www.hhs.gov/sites/default/files/surgeon-general-misinformation-advisory.pdf

National Institute for Health and Care Excellence. (2014 updated 2019, Feb 27). *Intrapartum care: Care of healthy women and their babies during childbirth: 2019 surveillance of intrapartum care for healthy women and babies (NICE guideline CG190).* https://www.nice.org.uk/guidance/cg190/resources/2019-surveillance-of-intrapartum-care-for-healthy-women-and-babies-nice-guideline-cg190-pdf-8701143147205

Nichols, T. R., Welborn, A., Gringle, M. R., & Lee, A. (2021). Social stigma and perinatal substance use services: Recognizing the power of the good mother ideal. *Contemporary Drug Problems, 48*(1), 19–37. https://doi.org/10.1177/0091450920969200

Noordam, R., Aarts, N., Verhamme, K., Sturkenboom, M., Stricker, B., & Visser, L. (2015, Jan 6). Prescription and indication trends of antidepressant drugs in the Netherlands between 1996 and

2012: A dynamic population-based study. *European Journal of Clinical Pharmacology, 71*, 369–375. https://doi.org/10.1007/s00228-014-1803-x

Nove, A., Friberg, I., de Bernis, L., McConville, F., Moran, A., Najjemba, M., ten Hoope-Bender, P., Tracy, S., & Homer, C. (2021). Potential impact of midwives in preventing and reducing maternal and neonatal mortality and stillbirths: A lives saved tool modelling study. *The Lancet Global Health, 9*(1), e24–e32. https://doi.org/10.1016/S2214-109X(20)30397-1

Ollove, M. (2016, August 15). *A Shortage in the Nation's Maternal Health Care.* Pew Charitable Trusts. https://www.pewtrusts.org/en/research-and-analysis/blogs/stateline/2016/08/15/a-shortage-in-the-nations-maternal-health-care

Poškienė, I., Vanagas, G., Kirkilytė, A., & Nadišauskienė, R. (2021). Comparison of vaginal birth outcomes in midwifery-led versus physician-led setting: A propensity score-matched analysis. *Open Medicine, 16*(1), 1537–1543. https://doi.org/10.1515/med-2021-0373

Pretzer, W. (n.d.). *Vital midwives: Merging modern medicine and West African traditions.* Smithsonian Institute. https://womenshistory.si.edu/herstory/health-wellness-work/object/vital-midwives

Razzaghi, H., Meghani, M., Pingali, C., Crane, B., Naleway, N., Weintraub, E., & Patel, S. (2021, June 18). COVID-19 vaccination coverage among pregnant women during pregnancy — Eight Integrated Health Care Organizations, United States, December 14, 2020–May 8, 2021. *Morbidity and Mortality Weekly Report, 70*(24), 895–899. https://doi.org/10.15585/mmwr.mm7024e2

Running-Bear, U., Beals, J., Novins, D., & Manson, S. (2016, Apr-June). Gender differences among Alaska Native people seeking alcohol withdrawal treatment. *Substance Abuse, 37*(2), 372–378. https://doi.org/10.1080/08897077.2015.1133473

Saccone, G., Florio, A., Aiello, F., Venturella, R., DeAngelis, M., Locci, M., & Sardo, A. (2020, May 7). Psychological impact of coronavirus disease 2019 in pregnant women. *American Journal of Obstetrics and Gynecology, 223*(2), 293–295. https://doi.org/10.1016/j.ajog.2020.05.003

Schultz, K., Ciwang, T., Breiler, G., Evans-Campbell, T., & Pearson, C. (2018, Oct 18). "They gave me life": Motherhood and recovery in a tribal community. *Substance Use and Misuse, 53*(12), 1965–1973. https://doi.org/10.1080/10826084.2018.1449861

Southwell, B., Wood, J., & Navar, A. (2020). Roles for health care professionals in addressing patient-held misinformation beyond fact correction. *American Journal of Public Health, 110*(S3), S288–S289. https://doi.org/10.2105/AJPH.2020.305729

Stone, S., Ernst, E., & Stapleton, S. (2017). The freestanding birth center: Evidence for change in the delivery of care to childbearing families. In B. Anderson, J. Rooks, & R. Barroso (Eds.), *Best practices in midwifery* (2nd ed., pp. 261–281). Springer.

Terplan, M., Kennedy-Hendricks, A., & Chisolm, M. (2015, Sept 20). Prenatal substance use: Exploring assumptions of maternal unfitness. *Substance abuse: Research and treatment, 9*(S2), 1–4. https://doi.org/10.4137/SART.S23328

Toquinto, S., Berglas, N., McLemore, M., Delgado, A., & Roberts, S. (2020). Pregnant women's acceptability of alcohol, tobacco, and drug use screening and willingness to disclose use in pre-natal care. *Women's Health Issues, 30*(5), 345–352. https://doi.org/10.1016/j.whi.2020.05.004

United Nations. (2019, July 11). *A human rights-based approach to mistreatment and violence against women in reproductive health services with a focus on childbirth and obstetric violence.* Advancement of women, 74th session, A/74/137-EN-pdf

Varney, H., & Thompson, J. (2015). *A history of midwifery in the United States: The midwife said fear not.* Springer. https://doi.org/10.1891/9780826125385

Wallace, M., Hovert, D., Williams, C., & Mendola, P. (2016). Pregnancy-associated homicide and suicide in 37 US states with enhanced pregnancy surveillance. *American Journal of Obstetrics and Gynecology, 215*(3), 364.e1. https://doi.org/10.1016/j.ajog.2016.03.040

Wiessinger, D., West, D., & Pitman, T. (2010). *The womanly art of breastfeeding* (8th ed.). Ballantine Books.

Williams, D. (2016). *How racism makes us sick.* TedTalk. https://www.ted.com/talks/david_r_williams_how_racism_makes_us_sick?language=en

Wong, S., Chow, K., Leung, T., Ng, W., Ng, T., & Shek, C. (2004). Pregnancy and perinatal out-comes of women with severe acute respiratory syndrome. *American Journal of Obstetrics and Gynecology, 191*(1), 292–297. https://doi.org/10.1016/j.ajog.2003.11.019

World Health Organization. (2019). *Delivered by women, led by men: A gender and equity analysis of the global health and social workforce*. WHO Human Resources for Health Observer Series No. 24. 9789241515 pdf.

Zheng, L., Li, H., & Zhang, H. (2021). Cohort study of use of the hands-and knees-position as the first approach to resolving shoulder dystocia and preventing neonatal birth trauma. *Gynecology and Obstetrics Clinical Medicine, 1*(3), 160–163. https://doi.org/10.1016/j.gocm.2021.08.001

Zinsser, L., Stoll, K., Wieber, F., Pehlke-Milde, J., & Gross, M. (2020). Changing behavior in pregnant women: A scoping review. *Midwifery, 85*, 102680. https://doi.org/10.1016/j.midw.2020.102680

Chapter 12
Survival Services for American Mothers

Jennifer W. Foster

12.1 Meeting Basic Needs for Maternal Health

Despite the many differences among Americans, everyone shares the same basic, physical needs to survive. We need food to nourish the body, clean water to drink, and shelter to protect us from harm, either from the extremes of weather, or the dangers of unsafe streets or neighborhoods. We need to breathe air free of contaminants. While every individual suffers when these basic needs are not met, fractures in securing the necessities of survival affect maternal health in additional ways. The natural course of healthy pregnancy and ongoing maternal health can be disrupted for mothers who are faced with poor nutrition, or toxic environmental exposures via air, water, or shelter. Poor long-term health among mothers affects the whole family.

For women with reasonably solid financial resources in the United States (USA), securing the necessities for a healthy pregnancy is obtainable. For women with few financial resources, securing these necessities can be challenging in myriad ways (Shrider et al., 2021). The social determinants of health (SDoH) bring much to bear on pregnancy and childbirth outcomes. As a nation, Americans value motherhood. There arc long-standing policies, reflected in a variety of federal and state-supported programs, to assist a mother with limited financial resources to achieve resources necessary for a healthy pregnancy. Yet, the reality of a woman's life circumstances determines how she navigates the challenges to obtaining basic survival services.

In the USA, access to the survival services for many women is usually not completely absent. Rather, they are of low quality. In this context, this chapter examines the effects of food, water, clean air, and shelter on maternal health in relationship to the SDoH. It provides examples of responses to the needs of mothers as a reflection of the core cultural values of practicality and action-orientation,

J. W. Foster (✉)
Emory University, Atlanta, GA, USA

© The Author(s), under exclusive license to Springer Nature Switzerland AG 2023
B. A. Anderson, L. R. Roberts (eds.), *Maternal Health and American Cultural Values*,
Global Maternal and Child Health, https://doi.org/10.1007/978-3-031-23969-4_12

12.2 Basic Necessities for Survival

12.2.1 Food

Securing, storing, preparing, and eating food is central to everyday life for everyone. Good nutrition is essential to maternal health, but how do pregnant women in the USA know what they need to eat during pregnancy? In agrarian times, most families worked on farms and nutritional wisdom was passed down through generations. Currently, few American women live on farms, and the reach of relatively cheap, but ultra-processed, food is vast.

Good nutrition in pregnancy and lactation has been extensively studied scientifically, and this information is widely available via the internet. The United States Food and Drug Administration (FDA) is a key source of information about maternal nutrition and specific foods to avoid during pregnancy, e.g., certain kinds of seafood and fish (FDA, 2021). Professional organizations, prestigious medical institutions, the government, and both not-for-profit and for-profit organizations provide information about good nutrition in pregnancy.

Almost all (98%) of adults in the USA own cell phones, and the majority (85%) own smartphones (Pew Research Center, 2021, April 7). In theory, all women in the USA could access information about good nutrition in pregnancy via innovative mobile phone applications (apps), such as the gratis, TEXT4BABY app, which sends texts regarding health, nutrition, and safety information for each phase of gestation, as well as appointment reminders for prenatal care (https://text4baby.org).

Diet quality seems to be more important than the amount of energy consumed during pregnancy. A study by Rohatgi et al. (2017) documented the degree to which pregnant women obtain their energy from ultra-processed foods. These foods contribute to the chronic conditions of obesity, hypertension, and diabetes (2017). The discordance between access to knowledge about healthy food for pregnancy and the availability of healthy food for pregnancy is often the result of the specific location where women live (Carrillo-Álvarez et al., 2021). Many of the neighborhoods where levels of poverty and racial segregation are high are food deserts. The United States Department of Agriculture defines a food desert as an urban area with no ready access within one mile to a store with fresh and nutritious food options. In rural America, a food desert is defined as 10 miles or more from the nearest market (Dutko et al., 2012). In 2021, it is estimated that approximately 19 million people, or 6.2% of the total population, had limited access to a supermarket or grocery store (Annie E. Casey Foundation, 2021).

The reasons for food deserts are multiple. Healthier foods (such as fresh fruits and vegetables) are perishable and expensive. Grocery store chains consider establishing a market in low-income neighborhoods as an investment risk or sometimes a philanthropic endeavor. There are transportation and supply chain challenges in many areas, exacerbated by the COVID-19 pandemic. Also, aggressive marketing, convenience, and popularity of fast-food restaurants give them a ubiquitous, highly visible presence in most areas. Sometimes, in a food desert, these convenience foods are the only food sources available within a reasonable distance. Moreover, fast food has become so embedded in the daily lives of many Americans that basic knowledge of what constitutes a balanced meal has become lost.

For example, I (JWF) recall taking a diet recall for a small group of pregnant adolescents during a prenatal class. These young women lived in a very low-income neighborhood. When asked what they ate in the previous 24 hours, one young mother said, "For lunch I had MacDonald's." Another responded, "I had Taco Bell for dinner." They were unable to identify any specific foods included in their meals.

Also, the cost of food is rising. Since 1974, the federal Special Supplemental Nutrition Program for Women, Infants, and Children (WIC) has provided food assistance to low-income pregnant and breastfeeding women and children under the age of five. The basic eligibility requirement is a family income below 185% of the established federal poverty level. In 2018 (latest data available), the Food and Nutrition Service of the Department of Agriculture estimates that 1.7 million infants (45% of all infants) born in the USA received WIC supplements. The coverage rate for pregnant women, however, was only 53% of all those eligible, and there is much variation among states (Department of Agriculture, 2018).

12.2.2   Water

Since the passage of the Safe Drinking Water Act in 1974, all public water systems in the USA are required by law to follow the regulations and standards of the United States Environmental Protection Agency (EPA). The EPA requires every water supplier in the USA to provide its customers with a Consumer Confidence report. Private wells, however, are not included in this requirement. The Consumer Confidence report gives information about the monitoring and reporting of unsafe levels of contaminants, with information about toxic contaminants, such as lead, nitrate, and arsenic (Centers for Disease Control and Prevention (CDC), n.d.). In addition, the World Health Organization (WHO) cautions that exposure of the general population to arsenic and other toxic chemicals in water is linked to skin lesions, cancer, cardiovascular disease, and diabetes. Exposure to clinical symptoms can be as short as five years (WHO, 2018). Many childbearing women, especially those living in poverty, have experienced many years of exposure, putting them at increased risk for poor maternal health outcomes.

In comparison to many nations, the USA has well-established safe, potable water. Many Americans take the safety of their water for granted. Data from the *Healthy People 2030* document reveals that in 2020, 93% of Americans received water that met the regulations of the Safe Drinking Water Act (Healthy People, 2030). The enforcement of the Safe Drinking Water Act is uneven, however. The National Resources Defense Council has reported that in 5000 community water systems, serving 27 million people, there have been over 12,000 health-based violations (Fedinick et al., 2017).

To appreciate the complexity and inequality in clean water enforcement, a detailed view of two, high-profile examples of gross water contamination is illustrative. One significant crisis occurred in Flint, Michigan in 2014; the aftermath continues to the present. The other crisis occurred in Honolulu, Hawaii in 2021; the full resolution is yet to be determined at the time of this writing.

12.2.2.1   Exemplar: Water in Flint, Michigan

The Flint River flows through the city of Flint, Michigan, the birthplace of General Motors. Despite an era when Flint was a prosperous town, for many years the river was used as a disposal for the treated and untreated waste from factories and meat plants, toxins from leached landfills, and raw sewage. For fifty years, the drinking water in Flint had been sourced from the Detroit River, not the Flint River. As automotive production declined in Flint, so too did the population. Many left Flint, but the poorest people remained. The majority are Black with about 45% of the population of Flint living below the poverty level (Denchak, 2018).

In 2011, the city of Flint went bankrupt, and the state took over the city management. In 2013, a cost-saving action was taken to cease using the Detroit River for drinking and to pump water temporarily from the Flint River until a pipeline could be built from Lake Huron. The Flint River water, while highly corrosive, was not treated. The lead in the water, highly toxic to children as well as undermining maternal health, leached out from the city's aging pipes (Denchak, 2018).

For over 18 months, nearly 9000 children were supplied with lead-contaminated water (Tanner, 2016). The switch to the Flint River coincided with an outbreak of Legionnaire's disease that killed 12 people and sickened many others because the city had not sufficiently chlorinated the water. When the city added more chlorine without addressing the other issues of the quality of the water, elevated levels of trihalomethane (TTHM) were discovered. TTHM is a carcinogenic by-product of the chlorination of water (Denchak, 2018).

12.2.2.2   Exemplar: Water in Pearl Harbor, Hawaii

In November 2021, in Honolulu, Hawaii, 14,000 gallons of jet fuel leaked from an underground USA military storage tank storage into the water supply serving the Joint Base Pearl Harbor-Hickam. This storage facility, in Ant Hill on the island of O'ahu, was built in 1940 and carved into basalt rock to protect it from enemy attack. The Navy reports the fuel stored in the Ant Hill tanks is critical for naval operations throughout the Indo-Pacific region. The fuel storage is located about 100 feet above O'ahu's main freshwater aquifer. The Navy's wells provide the water for drinking, cooking, bathing, and washing for 93,000 users (EPA, 2021).

In the spring of 2021, some families on the base began to notice a foul odor in the water, but it was not until December that the Hawaii Department of Health issued an emergency order, after Naval tests in November 2021 showed that the spilled fuel had contaminated a water well at Joint Base Pearl Harbor-Hickam. The order required the Navy to develop a plan that would empty the fuel tanks, identify needed repairs, address deficiencies, and install a water-treatment system at the contaminated well. In the midst of the COVID-19 pandemic, over 3500 military families were relocated to hotels over the Thanksgiving and Christmas holidays of 2021 (Britzky, 2022). The cost of lodging, transportation, and water cleansing for the exposed families was estimated to be about 250 million dollars (Horton, 2022).

12.2.3 Air

Research on air pollution and its negative impact on health is abundant (Lee et al., 2020), and there is good documentation about the higher-than-average air pollution exposures for racial/ethnic minority and low-income populations in the USA (Bowe et al., 2019). Low-income neighborhoods are more likely to experience high traffic noise, elemental carbon attributable to traffic (ECAT), and to be situated near facilities that emit particulate matter (PM). $PM_{2.5}$ is the threshold of tiny particles in the air that cause hazy air and reduced visibility. A study to quantify nationwide disparities in the location of particulate matter facilities found disproportionately high burdens of $PM_{2.5}$ for non-Whites and for those living in poverty. The disparity for Blacks was more pronounced than the disparity for all populations living in poverty (Mikati et al., 2018).

The reasons for the disparity in air pollution burden include, but are not limited to, the historical "redlining" of neighborhoods by the federally sponsored Homeowners' Loan Corporation. Beginning in the 1930s, neighborhoods were graded on a 4-point scale from A (most desirable) to D (hazardous – red-lined). Black and immigrant communities received a D rating and were typically ineligible for federally backed loans or favorable mortgage terms. Local governments chose to place hazardous and polluting industries in and near the red-lined D neighborhoods (Benjamins & De Maio, 2021; Lane et al., 2022; Liu et al., 2021).

Regarding maternal health, air pollution and birth outcomes have been the subject of a growing body of research. There is evidence that air pollution affects birth outcomes negatively, but the strength of the evidence depends on the outcome being examined (Sram et al., 2005; Shah & Balkhair, 2011). The preponderance of research on birth outcomes is focused on preterm birth, intrauterine growth restriction, and maternal exposures in early pregnancy associated with abnormal fetal lung development during organogenesis (Korten et al., 2017). These studies indicate, but do not sufficiently emphasize, the key link between maternal health and birth outcomes.

In pregnancy, the damaging effects of air pollution impact the maternal cardiovascular system. Exposure to toxic air raises blood pressure by interacting with the sympathetic nervous system, promoting oxidative stress and circulating cytokines, or altering the vascular endothelium (Hu et al., 2019). Increased maternal systolic blood pressure is associated with traffic (ECAT), especially when traffic is combined with other ambient noise (Sears et al., 2018). In addition to hypertensive disorders, a recent systematic review supported the hypothesis that there is an increased risk of maternal gestational diabetes with air pollution exposure. Oxidative stress and inflammation also promote insulin resistance (Hu et al., 2019). The association of $PM_{2.5}$ was specifically implicated in the development of gestational diabetes during preconception and the first two trimesters of pregnancy (Rammah et al., 2020).

12.2.4 Shelter

Survival depends on shelter, and shelter exists within the context of neighborhood. Public policy discourse related to housing recognizes three interconnected elements, the physical, the social, and the psychological. The physical is the obvious element, such as the location, population density, maintenance of housing, quality of building materials, sanitation and the prevalence of toxins (such as asbestos and lead), and the prevalence of pests (such as rats and roaches). The social element encompasses threats to safety, noise, social networks, and housing costs. The psychological element includes household conflicts and sense of permanence, especially if there are concerns about financial instability, stability of housing, or real or imagined threat of homelessness. All three of these interconnected elements affect health (Rauh et al., 2008).

While the positive association between safe, stable, affordable housing, and health has been established for quite some time, the complexity of the relationship between housing and maternal-infant health has been only recently explored. Maternal and infant health outcomes are poorer in racially segregated households. Racially segregated households have higher crime, poverty, and resource deprivation. Resource deprivation encompasses distance from access to quality food, such as food deserts, quality education, and healthcare. Racially segregated neighborhoods have higher rates of "physical incivilities," such as vacant housing, blight, litter, and graffiti (Reece, 2021).

Neighborhoods with high levels of economic deprivation are strongly associated with preterm birth (Messer et al., 2012). Preterm birth constitutes the greatest proportion of infant mortality, and with few exceptions, is contingent on maternal health. Moreover, in hyper-racially segregated areas, infants born to Black mothers had 50% higher preterm rates than infants born to White mothers. Additionally, Black infants in hyper-segregated areas were significantly more likely to be born preterm than compared with infants not from hyper-segregated areas (Osypuk & Acevedo-Garcia, 2008). Hypertensive disorders of pregnancy may lead to preterm birth. Additionally, stress hormones can initiate early labor and may depress maternal immune systems, leading to greater susceptibility to disease (Reece, 2021). Homeless women are more at risk for pregnancy complications (Clark et al., 2019), and housing instability is significantly associated with childbirth complications

(Ditosto et al., 2021). Maternal health outcomes are a function of neighborhood quality.

At the time of this writing, the USA is experiencing a housing shortage with insufficient units available for rent or purchase (Parrott & Zandi, 2021). This factor contributes to housing insecurity for many people. More American households are headed by renters than at any point since 1965 (Pew Research Center, 2017, July 19). Since the COVID-19 pandemic, rents have increased in some metropolitan areas more than 40% in a year, increasing housing insecurity, with its negative consequences on maternal health (Sainato, 2022, Feb 16).

12.3   Cultural Values and Survival

There is vast inequality in the context of mothers' lives in the USA depending upon the SDoH. Poverty and racial segregation create many hurdles for mothers to attain what they need, but the increase in housing insecurity is just one example to emphasize that even women not in poverty face environmental threats to survival basics. Faced with these environmental threats, many Americans embrace the cultural values of practicality and action-orientation in problem solving. Details about the cases discussed above in Flint, Michigan and Joint Base Pearl Harbor Hickam explain how citizens embody these values, often with mothers taking the lead.

12.3.1   Citizen Action in Flint

When the city of Flint went bankrupt, the state-appointed city manager took a decisive and practical cost-cutting action by shutting off the Detroit river as the source of water for Flint. He changed the water source to the Flint river, until another pipeline could be built. The city manager saw the opportunity to save five million dollars for the city. It seemed to be a quick, efficient, and practical step to help ease the city's fiscal crisis. Flint's aging pipes leached lead from corrosive chemicals in the Flint river, with immediate impact upon 9000 children. A group of Flint citizens and faith-based groups organized to take action.

During city council meetings, one activist brought a bottle filled with filthy water from the Flint River and thrust it in front of the television cameras. This bold action led to national awareness of the problem. Local citizens formed a coalition with the American Civil Liberties Union and the Natural Resources Defense Council petitioning the EPA to launch a federal response to the crisis. Later, they filed a lawsuit alleging violation of the Safe Water Act. The lawsuit was settled in 2017, requiring the city of Flint and the state of Michigan to replace Flint's lead and galvanized steel service lines within three years, while simultaneously providing support for filtered water, public education, and extensive tap water testing (Natural Resources Defense

Council, 2017). The settlement claims are in process as of this writing (Diaz, 2021, Dec 29).

While the city's water has greatly improved since the legal settlement and numerous activists have received national media attention, the aftermath of the Flint crisis left a deep distrust of government to act in good faith on their behalf (Centers for Disease Control and Prevention, n.d.). Ironically, although tap water in Flint is now much cleaner, few of the citizens of that city use it, choosing to buy bottled water instead. Too many people had suffered from associated physical ailments, e.g., skin rashes, pneumonia, strokes, and kidney damage. Some of those afflicted had no health insurance and incurred large medical bills. The psychological aftermath also caused substantial anxiety and panic attacks, even from simply hearing water running from the tap. There were so many miscarriages in Flint that University of Kansas economists reported a drop in fertility rate by 12%, and fetal death increase by 58% (Glenza, 2018). The impact on maternal health is unknown, although the link of toxic water to cardiovascular disease and diabetes, as described by the WHO (, 2018), is sobering in light of the high maternal mortality and morbidity among Black women, who comprise the majority of pregnant women in Flint.

12.3.2 Action of Citizen Soldiers and Military Families in Honolulu

In contrast to Flint, the population at the Joint Base Pearl Harbor Hickam were neither impoverished nor racially segregated. When the fuel tanks leaked into the water, sickening the children, as in Flint, the parents took action. Even after families on the base were provided with bottled water by the Navy, some of the children persisted with severe vomiting, diarrhea, and abdominal pain. Parents brought them to the military hospital's emergency department. Medical staff who evaluated the sick children explained that even if bottled water were used for drinking and cooking, utensils and linens washed with petroleum-contaminated water could still cause illness. The impact on the health of childbearing women with their use of utensils and linens washed in petroleum-contaminated water is unknown.

One mother exemplifies this parental action-orientation. As soon as this mother of a sick child learned from medical staff about ongoing exposure to contaminated water, she reported it to personnel at her child's daycare. This institution cared for over 200 children on the base. Yet, none of the daycare staff had been informed by Navy's leadership about utensils and linens as sources of contamination. This mother took action, communicating up the chain of command to her boss, and thereafter, to the chief staff officer for the Joint Base Pearl Harbor Hickam. She also wrote an open letter to the Secretary of Defense, including his wife on the communication (Britzky, 2022, March 7). This is an excellent example of the American cultural value of action-orientation implemented by one mother. By March 2022, the Secretary of Defense decided to close the Red Hill bulk fuel storage facility

(Britzky, 2022, March 7). Since the decision by the Secretary of Defense, concerned citizens of Honolulu have continued to keep the pressure on the Navy to immediately do whatever it takes to prevent future fuel leakage into Honolulu's aquifers. Prior to defueling the tanks, the Hawaii Department of Health issued an emergency order for the Navy to conduct an independent assessment of the current status of the tanks. The report indicated there were so many safety hazards that it could take two years to even ready the tanks for defueling (Jedra, 2022, May 27).

Less than two weeks after the Navy's (redacted) report by the independent consultant was made public, the news website, *Popular Resistance*, published an alternative option to transport the fuel through a smaller pipe system that would not take two years, but rather, could realistically take only 27 days if it were truly a priority. The author of the publication is a retired Army colonel (Wright, 2022, June 6). It is noteworthy that while there have been many concerned citizens who acted to pressure local government officials to respond to these two crises in water contamination, the key organizers of the citizenry in both cases were mothers with children. However, the impact of this toxic water on maternal health outcomes has still not been evaluated. In conversation with military activists, I (JWF) have learned the problem has not been resolved.

12.3.3   Citizen Response to Food Deserts and Food Waste

One action-oriented response to food deserts is the trend for community gardens (Department of Agriculture, n.d.). The Department of Agriculture defines community gardens as plots of land, usually in urban areas, that are rented by individuals or groups for private gardens or for the benefit of those caring for the garden (Department of Agriculture, 2022). One study of the impact of community gardens found that the frequency of participants' worries about food security before the gardening season was 31.2%, and after the gardening season was 3.1%. Eating vegetables "several times a day" before the gardening season went from 18.2% of those sampled to 84.8% after the gardening season (Carney et al., 2012).

Concerned citizens in America are increasingly aware of the juxtaposition of two food realities: there are food deserts in poor neighborhoods and there is tremendous food waste across the nation. ReFed, a philanthropic organization whose mission is to end food waste, provides data-driven solutions across the food system. In their mission statement, ReFed states, "It's action that can solve the food waste crisis" (ReFed.org. n.d.-a. About us, para 1). They estimate that 24% of all the food produced in the USA goes to waste (ReFed.org, Food waste challenge. n.d.-b).

The EPA catalogs projects and grantees across the nation who are working to reduce food waste. Across many communities, the organization of rapid response groups to redistribute excess food from restaurants and supermarkets is growing. For example, numerous cellphone applications have made it possible for those working with large volumes of edible but rejected food to alert food banks and food pantries to accept them, so that delivery drivers can immediately transfer the food to those sites. There are also apps to alert individual volunteers to pick up surplus food in restaurants and deliver directly to households in need (Bozhinova, 2018). Community organizers also have been working to convince discount stores in poor or isolated areas to sell sustainably sourced produce (Greenfield, 2019). All of these actions are examples of the cultural values of practicality and action-orientation. These actions help to provide food security for mothers in need.

12.3.4   Barriers to Reaping the Benefits of Citizen Action

If (almost) all mothers in America share the values of practicality and action-orientation, why would mothers *not* use innovative, practical, technical assistance designed to help them achieve maternal health? Why don't more mothers enroll in TEXT4BABY? Why do eligible mothers fail to enroll for the WIC program? Evaluation research of TEXT-4-BABY and other maternal health applications have revealed that even with free access to these applications, the uptake of health education is hindered when health literacy is low. *Healthy People 2030* defines health literacy as both personal (the degree to which individuals have the ability to find, understand, and use information and services to inform health-related decisions and actions) and organizational (the degree to which organizations equitably enable individuals to find, understand, and use information and services to inform health-related decisions and actions) (Healthy People 2030). Face-to-face support is lacking and needed (Gazmarian et al., 2014, Foster et al., 2015).

Despite the prevalence of cellphones, not all mothers have smartphones and their ability to pay for cell service on a consistent basis may be problematic. Failure to meet the payment schedule for cell phones may result in frequent changes in phone numbers, loss of apps, and dropped enrollment in services. The mother may need to re-enroll and low health literacy may become a barrier (Foster et al., 2015).

Nevertheless, practicality is at play in the decisions mothers make to secure food, even in food deserts. Frequenting a local fast-food restaurant or purchasing ultra-processed foods at the local convenience store is often much easier, more immediate, and more practical, especially when transportation is an issue. Driving a longer distance to find a healthier food source often requires using limited public transportation or access to an automobile with increasingly expensive gasoline.

12.3.5   Practicality: Necessary But Not Sufficient

While American's practicality and can-do attitude for those in need may demonstrate laudable values, it is unlikely that mothers in every circumstance will benefit from them. In comparison, there are many high-resource countries whose cultural values do not depend on philanthropic organizations or concerned citizens to help mothers in need. Rather, these countries have essentially unified political support for a strong, central government mandate to ensure health for all mothers, regardless of income.

All the Scandinavian countries and Iceland rank highest in their policy commitment to mothers and families (Rostgard, 2014). A number of European countries follow close behind (State of the World's Mothers, 2015). The non-governmental organization, *Save the Children,* rated Norway as the number one nation with measurable indices of caring for mothers. The Norwegian government gives lump sum grants to mothers for every child born. Childcare benefits are also paid monthly, regardless of income. Daycare centers are heavily subsidized, there is universal healthcare access, and parents are entitled to up to 20 days paid leave per year to care for a sick child. Working women in Norway can take nearly a year of maternity leave at full pay (Beglund, 2010, May 4). All of these policy measures support optimal maternal health outcomes in Norway. The USA is the only high-resource nation that does not guarantee paid leave to mothers after childbirth (Tikkanen et al., 2020).

12.4 Summary

Mothers in America, depending on their position relative to the SDoH, may have to overcome enormous hurdles to secure these basic survival services. Mothers in poverty and those who live in racially segregated areas are much more likely to struggle. These mothers are often the same population that has the worst maternal health, at times with disastrous outcomes during pregnancy, childbirth, the postpartum, or over the course of their lives with chronic illness, often untreated.

Concerned citizens across the nation have taken action to ameliorate the problems of food deserts, contaminated water, poor housing, and air pollution. Because Americans value practicality as well as action-orientation, the approaches to these problems are both innovative and technologically advanced. However, in contrast to other high-resource nations, the USA is not unified about the role of a strong central government approach in ensuring the health of *every* mother.

While it is unlikely that every mother in need will be reached, the cultural values of practicality and action-orientation motivate mothers. Those in poverty and without adequate resources do what is necessary, most convenient, and most practical even when not in the best interest of their own health. As a result, maternal health outcomes in the USA are highly variable and unequal.

References

Annie E. Casey Foundation. (2021). *Exploring America's food deserts.* https://www.aecf.org/blog/exploring-americas-food-deserts

Beglund, N. (2010, May 4). *Norway best in world for mothers.* https://www.newsinenglish.no/2010/05/04/norway-best-in-world-for-mothers/.

Benjamins, M. R., & De Maio, F. (2021). *Unequal cities: Structural racism and the death gap in America's largest cities.* Johns Hopkins University Press.

Bowe, B., Xie, Y., Yan, Y., & Al-Aly, Z. (2019). Burden of cause-specific mortality associated with $PM_{2.5}$ air pollution in the United States. *Journal of the American Medical Association, Network Open, 2*(11), e1915834. https://doi.org/10.1001/jamanetworkopen.2019.15834

Bozhinova, K. (2018). *Sixteen apps helping companies and consumers prevent food waste.* https://www.greenbiz.com/article/16-apps-helping-companies-and-consumers-prevent-food-waste.

Britzky, H. (2022, Jan 6). *Inside one Army family's struggle amid the Navy's water crisis in Hawaii.* https://taskandpurpose.com/news/navy-water-contamination-crisis-hawaii/

Britzney, H. (2022, March 7). *The Navy's Red Hill fuel storage facility is being shut down for good.* https://taskandpurpose.com/news/pentagon-navy-closing-red-hill-fuel-facility-hawaii/.

Carney, R., Hameda, J., Rdesinski, R., Sprager, L., Nichols, K., Liu, B. Y., Pelayo, J., Sanchez, M. A., & Shannon, J. (2012). Impact of a community garden program on vegetable intake, food security and family relationships: A community-based participatory research study. *Journal of Community Health, 37*(4), 874–881. https://doi.org/10.1007/s10900-011-9522-z

Carrillo-Álvarez, E., Salinas-Roca, B., Costa-Tutusaus, L., Milà-Villarroel, R., & Shankar Krishnan, N. (2021). The measurement of food insecurity in high-income countries: A scoping review. *International Journal of Environmental Research and Public Health, 18*, 9829. https://doi.org/10.3390/ijerph18189829

Centers for Disease Control and Prevention. Consumer Confidence Reports. (n.d.). https://www.cdc.gov/healthywater/drinking/public/understanding_ccr.html

Clark, R., Weinreb, L., Flahive, J., & Seifert, R. (2019). Homelessness contributes to pregnancy complications. *Health Affairs, 38*(1), 139–146. https://www.healthaffairs.org

Denchak, M. (2018). *Flint water crisis: Everything you need to know.* Natural Resources Defense Council. https://www.nrdc.org/stories/flint-water-crisis-everything-you-need-know#sec-summary.

Diaz, A. (2021, Dec 29). Flint water settlement claims to process to begin January 12, 2022. https://flintbeat.com/flint-water-settlement-claims-process-to-begin-jan-12-2022/

Ditosto, J., Holder, K., Soyemi, E., Beestrum, M., & Yee, L. (2021). Housing instability and adverse perinatal outcomes: A systematic review. *American Journal of Obstetrics and Gynecology MFM, 3*, 100477. https://www.ajogmfm.org/article/S2589-9333(21)00172-5/fulltext

Dutko, P., Ver Ploeg, M., & Farrigan, T. (2012, August). *Characteristics and influential factors of food deserts.* U.S. Department of Agriculture, Economic Research Service. https://www.ers.usda.gov/webdocs/publications/45014/30939_err140_reportsummary.pdf?v=8736.8

Fedinick, K. P., Wu, M., Panditheratne, M., & Olson, E. D. (2017). *Threats on tap: Widespread violations highlight need for investment in water infrastructure and protections.* Natural Resources Defense Council. https://www.nrdc.org/resources/threats-tap-widespread-violations-water-infrastructure

Foster, J., Miller, L., Isbell, S., Shields, T., Worthy, N., Dunlop, A., & L. (2015). mHealth to promote pregnancy and interconception health among African-American women at risk for adverse birth outcomes: A pilot study. *mHealth, 1*, 20. https://doi.org/10.3978/j.issn.2306-9740.2015.12.01

Gazmarian, J. A., Elon, L., Yang, B., Graham, M., & Parker, K. (2014). Text4baby program: An opportunity to reach underserved pregnant and postpartum women? *Maternal Child Health Journal, 18*, 223–232. https://doi.org/10.1007/s10995-013-1258-1

Glenza, J. (2018, April 25). *Flint crisis, four years on: What little trust is left continues to wash away.* The Guardian. https://www.theguardian.com/us-news/2018/apr/25/flint-water-crisis-four-years-later.

Greenfield, N. (2019). *From farms to Dollar Stores: One woman's fight for justice.* Natural Resources Defense Council. https://www.nrdc.org/stories/farms-dollar-stores-one-womans-fight-

Healthy People. (2030). U.S. Department of Health and Human Services, Office of Disease Prevention and Health Promotion. https://health.gov/healthypeople/objectives-and-data/social-determinants-health

Horton, A. (2022, January 11). *Pearl Harbor water contamination: Lawmakers scold Navy over Hawaii health crisis.* The Washington Post. https://www.washingtonpost.com/national-security/2022/01/10/pearl-harbor-water-contamination/

Hu, C.-Y., Gao, X., Fang, Y., Jiang, W., Huang, K., Hua, X.-G., Yang, X.-J., Chen, H.-B., Jiang, X., & Zhang, X.-J. (2019). Human epidemiological evidence about the association between air pollution exposure and gestational diabetes mellitus: A systematic review and meta-analysis. *Environmental Research.* https://doi.org/10.1016/j.envres.2019.108843,180

Jedra, C. (2022, May 27). Consultant: Fixing Red Hill's decrepit infrastructure could take 2 years. Honolulu Civil Beat. https://www.civilbeat.org/2022/05/consultant-fixing-red-hills-decrepit-infrasturcture-could-take-2 years/

Korten, I., Ramsey, K., & Latzin, P. (2017). Air pollution in pregnancy and lung development in the child. *Pediatric Respiratory Reviews, 21*, 38–46. https://doi.org/10.1016/j.prrv.2016.08.008

Lane, H., Morello-Frosch, R., Marshall, J. D., & Apte, J. S. (2022). Historical redlining is associated with present-day air pollution disparities in U.S. cities. *Environmental and Technology Letters*, American Chemical Society. https://doi.org/10.1021/acs.estlett.1c01012.

Lee, K. K., Bing, R., Kiang, J., Bashir, S., Spath, N., Stelzle, D., Mortimer, K., Bularga, A., Doudesis, D., Joshi, S. S., Strachan, F., Gumy, S., Adair-Rohani, H., Attia, E. F., Chung, M. H., Miller, M. R., Newby, D. E., Mills, N. L., McAllister, D. A., & Shah, A. S. (2020). Adverse health effects associated with household air pollution: A systematic review: Meta-analysis, and burden estimation study. *Lancet Global Health, 8*(11), e1427–e1434. https://doi.org/10.1016/S2214-109X(20)30343-0

Liu, J., Clark, L. P., Bechle, M. J., Hajat, A., Kim, S. Y., Robinson, A. L., Sheppard, L., Szpiro, A. A., & Marshall, J. D. (2021). Disparities in air pollution exposure in the United States by race/ethnicity and income, 1990-2010. *Environmental Health Perspectives, 129*(12), 127005. https://doi.org/10.1289/EHP8584

Messer, L., Vinikoor-Imler, L. C., & Laraia, B. (2012). Conceptualizing neighborhood space: Consistency and variation of associations for neighborhood factors and pregnancy health across multiple neighborhood units. *Health & Place, 18*(4), 805–813. https://doi.org/10.1016/j.healthplace.2012.03.012

Mikati, I., Benson, A., Luben, T., Sacks, J., & Richmond -Bryant, J. (2018). Disparities in distribution of particulate matter emission sources by race and poverty status. *American Journal of Public Health, 108*, 480–485. https://doi.org/10.2105/AJPH.2017.304297

Natural Resources Defense Council. (2017). *Flint, Michigan safe drinking water lawsuit settlement.* Natural Resources Defense Council. https://www.nrdc.org/resources/flint-mi

Osypuk, T., & Acevedo-Garcia, D. (2008). Are racial disparities in preterm birth larger in hypersegregated areas? *American Journal of Epidemiology, 167*(11), 1295–1304. https://doi.org/10.1093/aje/kwn043

Parrott, J., & Zandi, M. (2021, March). *Overcoming the nation's daunting housing supply shortage.* Moody Analytics. https://www.moodysanalytics.com/-/media/article/2021/Overcoming-the-Nations-Housing-Supply-Shortage.pdf

Pew Research Center. (2017, July 19). *More U. S. Households are renting than at any point in 50 years.* Pew Research Center. https://www.pewresearch.org/fact-tank/2017/07/19/more-u-s-households-are-renting-than-at-any-point-in-50-years/

Pew Research Center. (2021, April 7). *Demographics of mobile device ownership and adoption in the United States.* Pew Research Center. https://www.pewresearch.org/internet/fact-sheet/mobile/.

Rammah, A., Whitworth, K. W., & Symanski, E. (2020). Particle air pollution and gestational diabetes in Houston, Texas. *Environmental Research, 190.* https://doi.org/10.1016/j.envres.2020.109988

Rauh, V., Landrigan, P., & Claudio, L. (2008). Intersection of poverty and environmental exposures. *Annals of New York Academy of Sciences, 1136*, 276–288. https://doi.org/10.1196/annals.1425.032

Reece, J. (2021). More than shelter: Housing for urban maternal and infant health. *International Journal of Environmental Research and Public Health, 18*, 3331. https://doi.org/10.3390/ijerph18073331

ReFed. (n.d.-a). About us. https://refed.org/about/who-we-are/

ReFed. (n.d.-b). Food waste challenge. https://refed.org/food-waste/the-challenge/#overview

Rohatgi, K. W., Tinius, R. A., Cade, W. T., Steele, E. M., Cahill, A. G., & Parra, D. C. (2017). Relationships between consumption of ultra-processed foods, gestational weight gain and neonatal outcomes in a sample of US pregnant women. *Peer Journal, 5*, e4091. https://doi.org/10.7717/peerj.4091

Rostgard, T. (2014). *Family policies in Scandinavia.* https://library.fes.de/pdf-files/id/11106.pdf

Sainato, M..(2022, Feb 16). Renters across US face sharp increases-averaging up to 40% in some cities. (2022, Feb 16). *The Guardian.* https://www.theguardian.com/us-news/2022/feb/16/renters-rent-increases-us-lease

Sears, C. G., Braun, J. M., Ryan, P. H., Xu, Y., Werner, E. F., Lanphear, B. P., & Wellenius, G. A. (2018). The association of traffic-related air and noise pollution with maternal blood pressure and hypertensive disorders of pregnancy in the HOME study cohort. *Environment International, 574-581*, 574. https://doi.org/10.1016/j.envint.2018.09.049

Shah, P., & Balkhair, T. (2011). Air pollution and birth outcomes: A systematic review. *Environment International, 37*, 498–516. https://doi.org/10.1016/j.envint.2010.10.009

Shrider, E. A., Kollar, M., Chen, F., & Semega, J. (2021). *Income and poverty in the United States: 2020. U.S. Census Bureau, current population reports: 60–273, U.S.* Government Publishing Office. https://cps.ipums.org/cps/resources/poverty/PovReport20.pdf

Sram, R., Binkova, B., Dejmek, J., & Bobak, M. (2005). Ambient air pollution and pregnancy outcomes: A review. *Environmental Health Perspectives, 113*(4), 375–382.

State of the World's Mothers. (2015). *Save The Children.* Retrieved from https://www.savethechildren.net/state-worlds-mothers-2015

Tanner, K. (2016, January 16). *All Flint's children must be treated as exposed to lead.* Detroit Free Press https://www.freep.com/story/opinion/contributors/raw-data/2016/01/16/map-8657-flints-youngest-children-exposed-lead/78818888/.

TEXT4BABY. (n.d.). Free text messages to keep you and your baby healthy. https://text4baby.org

Tikkanen, R., Gunja, MZ., Fitzgerald, M., & Zephyrin, L. (2020). Maternal mortality and maternal care in the United States compared to 10 other developed countries. Commonwealth Fund. https://www.commonwealthfund.org/publications/issue-briefs/2020/nov/maternal-mortality-maternity-care-us-compared-10-countries

United States Department of Agriculture. (2018). WIC eligibility and coverage rates – 2018. https://www.fns.usda.gov/wic/eligibility-and-coverage-rates-2018.

United States Department of Agriculture. (2022). Wasted food programs and resources across the United States. https://www.epa.gov/sustainable-management-food/wasted-food-programs-and-resources-across-united-states

United States Department of Agriculture. (n.d.). Community gardening. https://www.nal.usda.gov/legacy/afsic/community-gardening

United States Environmental Protection Agency. (2021). *Drinking water emergency at Joint Base Pearl Harbor-Hickam.* Honolulu. https://www.epa.gov/red-hill/drinking-water-emergency-joint-base-pearl-harbor-hickam-honolulu-hawaii-november-2021

United States Food and Drug Administration. (2021). Food safety for pregnant women and their unborn babies. https://www.fda.gov/food/people-risk-foodborne-illness/food-safety-booklet-pregnant-women-their-unborn-babies-and-children-under-five.

World Health Organization. (2018, Feb 15). Fact sheets: Arsenic. https://www.who.int/news-room/fact-sheets/detail/arsenic.

Wright, A. (2022, June 6). Emptying the Navy's Red Hill fuel tanks need not take 2 years. Popular Resistance. https://popularresistance.org/emptying-the-navys-red-hill-jetfuel-tanks-need-not-take-two-years/

Chapter 13
Community Influences on Maternal Safety

Mary de Chesnay

13.1 Individualism and Maternal Safety

Americans take great pride in the cultural value of individualism, a cultural strength enabling people to feel free to realize their dreams and goals. Freedom is prized. Autonomy is cherished. American children are taught that they can strive to be anything they want to be, even growing up to be the President of the nation. Many Euro-Americans tend to attribute outcomes to individual hard work and personal responsibility in contrast to some members of American sub-cultures who may attribute outcomes to fate or the result of social group activity (Fischer, 2008; Gorodnichenko & Roland, 2021). Individualism is particularly engrained in the traditions of predominately White Americans who claim to be descended from early pioneers or recent immigrants without strong ties to their countries of origin. Black and early Latinx immigrants seem to have more a sense of collectivism due to being enslaved or marginalized culturally or coming from cultures valuing interdependence. The cultural view of rugged American male individualism has also influenced gender discrimination as exemplified by the battle to codify the 19th Amendment on women's suffrage in 1920. Financial autonomy for women did not occur until the passage of the Equal Credit Opportunity Act in 1974 enabling women to obtain credit in their own names, although men already had the autonomy to do so (Abzug, 1974).

There is a delicate balance between individualism and disregard for the rights and needs of others. For some people, individualism equates to doing whatever they wish, regardless of their effect on others. For example, during the pandemic, while masks and social distance were mandated, and later, when vaccines were freely available, some people argued that they had a right not to comply, that the pandemic

M. de Chesnay (✉)
Kennesaw State University, Kennesaw, GA, USA

© The Author(s), under exclusive license to Springer Nature Switzerland AG 2023   167
B. A. Anderson, L. R. Roberts (eds.), *Maternal Health and American Cultural Values*,
Global Maternal and Child Health, https://doi.org/10.1007/978-3-031-23969-4_13

was not serious, and the measures to protect public health were unnecessary. Some became violent and abusive or mocked those who did comply. Some parents railed against protective mandates in public schools. Even some celebrities and athletes, as cultural heroes, contributed to this problem. While team sports are promoted as collaborative, individual "stars" are glorified, their messages heeded, scientifically correct or not. This tendency became particularly troubling during the COVID-19 pandemic with widespread misinformation and disinformation about the COVID-19 vaccine.

Autonomy coupled with a sense of personal responsibility can enhance social interdependence rather than promote conflict (Waterman, 1981). For example, during the mask mandate, those who chose to comply did so not only to protect themselves, but also perhaps because they accepted personal responsibility for the health of others. Individualism without collaboration with others and personal responsibility leads to social conflict, endangering vulnerable populations, including childbearing mothers. The multicultural environment within the USA, as well as the stresses of in the global economy, further point to the need for a balance between autonomy and interdependence (Xie & Lou, 2022).

While maternal safety and health outcomes are defined by physiological indicators, such as sepsis, bleeding, blood clots, and hypertension (Arnolds et al., 2019; Bernstein et al., 2017; MacDorman et al., 2021; Shields et al., 2015; Turner, 2019), they are equally framed by the social determinants of health (SDoH) as defined in *Healthy People 2030* (Healthy People 2030, n.d.) This chapter focuses on maternal health outcomes which are highly correlated to safe environments, one of the SDOH. This includes threats such as intimate partner violence that escalates when a woman becomes pregnant or living in a violent neighborhood. Opposition to gun laws and the perceived right to bear arms without adequate restraint increases environmental risk to vulnerable populations including mothers. Human trafficking is a threat in and outside the home. Vulnerability to human trafficking often begins in the home. Child sexual abuse is the strongest single predictor for sex trafficking in both girls and boys (Boyce et al., 2018; Ernewein & Nieves, 2015; Kennedy et al., 2021; Middleton et al., 2022; Reid et al., 2017). Isolation further heightens safety issues. American Indian and Alaska Native (AI/AN) mothers living in remote rural communities not only experience sexual assault at a higher rate than the general population (Murphy-Oikonen et al., 2021) but also, often disappear without a trace (Ficklin et al., 2021; Joseph, 2021). Systemic racism continues to pose safety risks especially for mothers of color. Compounding the safety issue is that their stories often go unheard, or are not believed by law enforcement when they try to tell their stories (Murphy-Oikonen et al., 2021).

Prevalent factors that affect maternal safety and health outcomes in the USA include intimate partner violence, lack of neighborhood security, access to weapons in public and private spaces, and human trafficking. These factors are discussed in terms of how they demonstrate the impact of individualism on maternal safety. The case studies are composite stories that describe risks to maternal safety when the mother has limited autonomy to make decisions.

13.2 Intimate Partner Violence and Maternal Safety

Several forms of intimate partner violence (IPV) are relevant to the topic of maternal safety. Generally, these are psychological, physical, and sexual. Bullying is an example of psychological violence such as threats to hurt or maim the mother, her other children, or her pets. Physical violence takes many forms, from slapping or pushing to beatings so severe that they result in serious injury to the mother, fetal death, murder, or murder-suicide. A special risk occurs in violent environments where gang members *pimp* (sexually trafficked) girls and women, including pregnant ones, within the gang. The woman's romantic partner may use violence to force compliance (Twis et al., 2020). Finally, sexual violence is represented by marital rape, defined as force and penetration without consent. All women are at risk, but indigenous mothers suffer higher rates of abuse by partners as well as sexual assault by strangers (Joseph, 2021; Le May, 2018; Mantegani, 2021; Murphy-Oikonen et al., 2021).

In a systematic review of IPV prevalence in the nations within the Americas, it was found that both physical and sexual violence is widespread from former or current partners (Bott et al., 2019). In a systematic review of longitudinal studies, the strongest risk factors for IPV were unplanned pregnancy and having parents with less than a high school education, suggesting the role of poverty as a SDoH influencing IPV (Yakubovich et al., 2018). Results of IPV include significant health risks, including depression and post-partum depression (Bacchus et al., 2018). Although the COVID-19 pandemic is too recent to make meaningful conclusions about change in prevalence of IPV, there is sufficient anecdotal evidence to suggest that the physiological effects of the virus and the psychological effects of pandemic restrictions are only part of the story and that increased rates of IPV will exacerbate those effects (Bettinger-Lopez & Bro, 2020; Malik & Naeem, 2020). There are also anecdotal stories from women who experienced increased IPV during the pandemic business closures when many lost their jobs.

13.2.1 Withholding Resources

One of the most effective ways that abusers, generally male partners, control pregnant and parenting mothers is by severely limiting access to resources. An abuser might give the mother enough to buy groceries, but not enough to enable her to save for her escape, especially if she has children and pets to protect. One common scenario is that during courtship, he convinces her to give up her job or education because he will take care of her. This technique is effective for women who were abused as children and are vulnerable to a continued cycle of abuse, or women who envision a life of staying home as a full-time wife and mother. He then isolates her from her family and friends so there is no one to provide resources. Even if she still had contacts with family and friends, she might be too ashamed to confide in them and ask for help (Bacchus et al., 2018; Yakubovich et al., 2018).

13.2.2 Threatening with Weapons

The prevalence of guns in American homes places abused mothers at special risk, especially if the partner drinks or uses drugs. Although there is little in the way of research on teen domestic violence, it is clear that the prevalence of guns in homes and the high rate of gun violence by teenagers create a unique blend of risk factors, including for pregnant adolescents (Bender et al., 2020; Goodyear et al., 2020). A retrospective study conducted in Philadelphia revealed that of over 35,000 incidents of IPV reported to police, almost 80% involved a batterer using a gun to threaten, pistol-whip, or shoot his victim (Sorenson & Schut, 2018).

13.2.3 Sexual Violence

Sexual violence is distinguished from physical violence in IPV. Though males can be victims, most victims are women and rape in the statutes names women as victim (Banerjee & Rao, 2022). Marital rape was only considered illegal across the USA since 1993 when it became banned in all 50 states. Prior to that, English common law prohibited a woman from charging her husband with rape, a centuries-old scourge of marriage (Banerjee & Rao, 2022). Still, many do not support mothers who try to report it (Bennice et al., 2019). Outcomes of sexual violence are maternal depression, gynecological problems from trauma, and a variety of physical health symptoms (Chen et al., 2020).

13.2.4 Taking Pets Hostage

There is a direct link between animal abuse and IPV with abusers often intentionally causing pain and suffering to the pet in order to control the mother. Some states have passed laws that allow for pets to be considered under the domestic violence definition in statutes and they are included in protection orders against the abuser (Blaney et al., 2021). Victims report being afraid to leave the abuser, putting up with the violence against themselves because they have nowhere to go with their pets and cannot afford to board them (Campbell et al., 2018; Geisbrecht, 2021).

An increasing number of shelters nationwide are willing to make arrangements for pets, either in domestic violence shelters or in local rescues (Stevenson et al., 2017). In Phoenix, Arizona, the Sojourner Center operates a Pet Companion Shelter where animals receive stress reduction and social enrichment. The shelter has a family visitation room for owners to spend quality time with their pets (Sojourner Center, 2022). Another Arizona organization, in collaboration with the Humane Society of the United States, connects IPV victims with several local foster placement organizations (Arizona Pet Project, 2022).

Box 13.1 Stranded: A Life Course Story of Intimate Partner Violence
He was so considerate when we were dating. He showered me with attention and took me to the best restaurants. He bought me beautiful clothes and presents. No one had ever done that for me. Then gradually after the wedding he changed. He controlled everything from the money to who I could see. I was not allowed to be with my family on holidays even when my father was dying. He hit me for everything- if I folded the towels wrong, if I forgot to close the blinds, when he did not like what I cooked. If I answered the phone, he demanded every detail and if it was a telemarketer he accused me of cheating on him and beat me.

One night I had the flu and tried to say "no" to sex. He forced himself on me so roughly that I hurt for days. I thought a baby would make him happy but instead it got worse when I was pregnant. Once he hit me in the stomach and I thought I lost the baby. When the baby came he was jealous of everything I did for her. My sister told me to leave, but how could I? He said if I ever left him, he would kill me, the baby, my cat, and my whole family. I had no money, no job, no education, no place to go. Even if I did go, I couldn't leave my cat behind because the shelters don't take animals. I felt like I had lost all my choices and freedom.

This story challenges textbook explanations of maternal outcomes. It causes us to listen more deeply for tales of sacrifice, grace, and the value of linked lives embedded in the life course of mothers.

13.3   Neighborhood Security

A mother can be at risk at home or outside the shelter of her home. Security can be an issue in the wellbeing of mothers in neighborhoods assumed to be safe in safe neighborhoods as well as in high crime areas. Gangs and criminal activity occur in both low-income and affluent areas. Home invasions are prevalent in all kinds of neighborhoods. Affluent residents have more valuables to steal but also more financial resources to create a safe environment.

Neighborhood environments play a critical role in maternal safety and health. Safe neighborhoods promote social interaction and interdependency within a climate of security. Unsafe environments create anxiety and fear of violence outside the home. High crime rates increase stress during pregnancy, negatively affect healthy behaviors, for instance, considering whether or not the neighborhood is a safe place to walk can affect a mother's decision about exercise. Thus the environment can contribute to adverse physiological effects like hypertension during childbearing. The air quality and the health of buildings (e.g., prevalence of toxic mold) are also critical factors (Laraia et al., 2007; Mayne et al., 2018; Shah et al., 2021; Shannon et al., 2020; Stanhope et al., 2021).

13.3.1 Individualism and Gun Safety in the Neighborhood

A clear example of the American cultural tension with individualism is the right to carry guns versus the safety of the public. Almost any object can be used as a weapon, but the national conversation generally revolves around guns. While handguns were previously the weapon of choice in mass shootings, assault weapons have been increasing in popularity (Schildkraut, 2019).

On one side of the argument are the Second Amendment defenders who argue from an absolute position, that they have the unlimited right to bear arms and oppose restrictions, such as improved background checks. The Second Amendment was originally crafted to ensure a well-armed militia. The National Rifle Association (NRA) wields lobbying power in supporting the right to bear arms. On the other side are advocates seeking to abolish all gun ownership. The anti-gun activists were particularly active in Georgia in the 1970s. While these advocates were protesting the position of the NRA, the city of Kennesaw in Georgia enacted legislation mandating every homeowner to own a gun, although it is not strictly enforced (Bozeman et al., 2006).

Mothers, as frequent victims of IPV and neighborhood assaults, are at particular risk in a culture of gun violence. In light of the many rogue killings of the American population, there is increasing support among the public across the political spectrum for stricter gun background checks both in the home and in the neighborhood. There is strong support for commonsense gun control legislation, identification of those at high risk for violence, and limiting the type of gun available for purchase. Among gun owners, 82% support enhanced criminal background checks. Even NRA members (74%) support required criminal background checks (Everytown for Gun Safety, n.d.; Spitzer, 2020). Many Americans, especially those personally affected by mass shootings, have called for better background checks on domestic abusers, the mentally ill, and people with a past history of violent behavior (Newman & Hartman, 2017). An exemplar follows.

Box 13.2 Unsafe in Our Own Neighborhood

One night my son, his baby sister, and I were all sitting on our front stoop with my baby girl. It was a hot summer night and the baby was sick. I needed to cool her off because there was no air conditioning in our building and my fan broke down. He saw a car coming slowly up the street and tried to hustle us inside. He said they were gang members. I was reaching for the baby when the first shots came. They missed me and my boy but three bullets killed my baby. She was only two years old. We have no freedom here.

This story challenges textbook explanations of maternal outcomes. It causes us to listen more deeply for tales of sacrifice, grace, and the value of linked lives embedded in the life course of mothers.

13.3.2 Maternal Mental Health in Unsafe Environments

The social environment in the neighborhood is related to mental health and depression. If a mother experiences fear, anxiety, and depression from living in an unsafe neighborhood, she lives in a state of constant worry for herself and her children. For instance, she may need to make hard decisions about how much and under what circumstances to allow her children to play outside (Assari et al., 2020; Choi et al., 2021; Diaz & Whitaker, 2013). In a study of neighborhood safety and social involvement, Black and White mothers rated neighborhood safety according to their self-reported levels of depression as well as what methods they used to discipline their children. Inadequate neighborhood safety was associated with maternal depression and harsh methods of discipline (Hill & Herman-Stahl, 2002).

A new twist on the environmental influence on maternal health is the restricted healthcare access legislation beginning with the Texas abortion law in 2021. By reducing or eliminating access to healthcare and restricted legal mobility, it is expected that three particularly vulnerable populations—pregnant adolescents, mothers without resources for mobility, and disabled mothers—are at enhanced risk for adverse maternal health outcomes (Gordon et al., 2022; Simpson, 2021).

13.3.3 Project Safe Neighborhoods

In 2001, the federal government launched a program to bring together multiple stakeholders to address violent crime in local communities. Coordinated by United States Attorney Offices in the 50 states and the territories, the project was designed to build trust, enhance enforcement, and support community-based organizations to build safer neighborhoods. The project included initiatives aimed at preventing and combatting crimes against mothers and children. In 2021, the violent crime reduction strategy was launched. They report some progress such as better enforcement in the control of illegal drugs and gun regulations (United States Department of Justice, 2022).

13.4 Human Trafficking and Maternal Safety

Human trafficking takes several forms: sex trafficking, baby trafficking, forced labor, organ trafficking, child marriage, and child soldiers. Human trafficking has serious adverse effects on both mental and physical health (Kaplan et al., 2018; Recknor et al., 2019). Reliable data on the extent of human trafficking do not exist because it is largely a crime hidden from view with traffickers going to great lengths to disguise their victims and keep their business private. Probably at least 25 million adults and children are exploited into forced labor or sex trafficking worldwide generating profits of $150 billion (White House, 2022). In line with the focus in this chapter on maternal safety and autonomy in decision-making, the discussion of human trafficking here will be limited to the links with intimate partner violence and missing and murdered indigenous mothers.

13.4.1 Impact of Sex Trafficking on Maternal Health

It is a misperception that sex trafficking is something that happens far away or that family members would never exploit their own children or partners. Not only are both statements false, but they allow exploitation to flourish. In the case study presented here, the young woman was "rescued" from an abusive situation at home by a pimp, who inserted himself into her life as a romantic partner and quickly became her new nightmare. Often trafficked women pregnant and contract sexually transmitted diseases. Studying data in a Midwestern city for the years 2008–2017, researchers found 59 cases where an intimate partner used physical and sexual violence against the trafficked victim (Koegler et al., 2020).

The internet provides easy marketing and perpetuates the view of women and girls as sex objects. Young girls in the sex trade experience high levels of violence from pimps and *johns* (men who solicit sex with prostitutes) as well as adverse mental and physical health effects, such as unplanned pregnancies and multiple unsafe abortions (Collins & Skarparis, 2020). These adverse effects spill over into the next generation of their children of who end up in the welfare system, if they survive (Stoklosa et al., 2022). For women who choose abortion or have it imposed upon them, the physical effects are as damaging as the mental health effects. One of my (MdC) psychotherapy clients was forced into a coat-hanger abortion even though abortion was legal. She explained that her partner (pseudo-husband who turned into a pimp) did not want to spend the money for a clinic so he used a coat hanger. She eventually escaped but was rendered permanently infertile.

13.4.2 Missing and Murdered American-Indian and Alaska Native Mothers

Little attention has been given to the special vulnerabilities of American Indian and Alaska Native (AI/AN) women who disappear and/or who are found murdered at an alarming rate (Hunt, 2021; Le May, 2018). In 2018, the Urban Indian Health Institute published data from 71 US cities to assess numbers across the nation (Lucchesi & Echo-Hawk, 2018). Researchers found 5712 cases reported in 2016 but these are likely a vast underestimate of the total number due to poor law enforcement databases and failure to track and report cases. What is clear is that AI/AN women, among them pregnant and parenting mothers, suffer high rates of domestic violence, sexual assault, and kidnapping into human trafficking rings (Joseph, 2021; Mantegani, 2021; Murphy-Oikonen et al., 2021). A report to the Minnesota

Legislature found that in Minnesota alone, while indigenous women make up only 1% of the state's population, they represent 8% of those who disappear. Between 2012 and 2020, in any given month, 27–54 American Indian women were missing (Martin-Rogers & Pendleton, 2020).

The explanation for these high rates of sexual violence is explained by a multitude of factors, beginning with the long-term effects of colonialism (Ficklin et al., 2021). Today, isolation, discrimination, poverty, alcoholism, and a history of genocide play a role in the perpetration of violence toward AI/NA mothers. Trapped in dangerous situations, lack of access to transportation in rural areas may force them to hitchhike, furthering compounding risk from persons with criminal intent (Morton, 2016). Survival sex may result in dangerous situations of childbearing (Sharma et al., 2021). The following case study is an exemplar.

Box 13.3 Enslaved and Betrayed: An Adolescent Mother Tells Her Story

I was 10 and my mother was working night shift when my stepfather started crawling into my bed at night. I never told my mother because he said it would hurt my mother to know he loved me more than her. I endured his threats and this abuse for three years before I took a bus across the country. At a bus stop, I met a man who was kind to me. He took me to dinner and arranged a hotel room so I wouldn't have to sleep on the street. I cried on his shoulder and told him my story. He seemed to care about me. Soon I agreed to have sex and he promised me a future of happiness – we would marry and have a family.

But, he explained, first he had to get out of debt, He told me if I loved him I would help him which would mean "dating" other men for money who demanded sex. A few months later I got pregnant and asked him when we would get married. Instead, he said he wasn't the baby's father and then I watched as he accepted money for me from another man. That man, whose name I never learned, insisted that I continue the pregnancy. I was not sure who was the father of the baby at this point.

When I started labor, he dumped me at a hospital. I had a long and painful birth, but when my little girl was born, I felt love for her, just wanting to hold her and take care of her. A few hours after the birth, he came to the hospital, telling the health providers he came to see his baby and his "wife." While he was holding the baby, he walked out of the hospital with the baby in his arms. The next day I was discharged. I gave the social worker the address of his apartment as my "home" and since I had nowhere else to go, I walked over there hoping to find my baby. He was there but no baby. There were men in the apartment with him and they paid him to have sex with me. I was only 14, raw from the birth. He walked out and left me alone with them.

The men got drunk and I escaped from the apartment. I called the social worker who met me right away. I was placed in foster care. The baby's "father" was never found and the social worker told me she thought the baby had been sold. I had been a sexual slave without any choices and I never saw my baby again.

This story challenges textbook explanations of maternal outcomes. It causes us to listen more deeply for tales of sacrifice, grace, and the value of linked lives embedded in the life course of mothers.

Sexual trafficking is one of the most dangerous threats to safety, maternal health, and survival. This adolescent survived but not without significant threats to her wellbeing. Her autonomy and ability to make decisions about herself and her baby were stolen from her.

13.5 Summary

This chapter highlights the cultural value of individualism as a factor influencing maternal safety and health outcomes. It explored the influence of this cultural value in the context of the SDoH of economic stability, education, healthcare access, and the neighborhood environment. A foundational and positive cultural value, individualism can promote and enhance maternal safety and health outcomes for many mothers. In the context of risks to safety, such as IPV, neighborhood violence, threats from deadly weapons, and sexual trafficking, the mother loses her ability to exercise individualism and autonomy.

References

Abzug, B. (1974). H.R.8163 equal credit opportunity act of 1974. https://www.congress.gov/bill/93rd-congress/house-bill/8163

Arizona Pet Project. (2022). About us. Arizona Pet Project, https://azpetproject.org/

Arnolds, D., Smith, A., Banayan, J., Holt, R., & Scavone, B. (2019). National partnership for maternal safety recommended early warning criteria are associated with maternal morbidity. *Anesthesia and Analgesia, 6*, 1621–1626.

Assari, S., Boyce, S., Caldwell, C., Bazargan, M., & Mincy, R. (2020). Family income and gang presence in the neighborhood: Diminished returns of Black families. *Urban Science, 4*(2), 1–11.

Bacchus, L. J., Ranganathan, M., Watts, C., & Devries, K. (2018). Recent intimate partner violence against women and health: A systematic review and meta-analysis of cohort studies. *BMJ Open, 8*(7), e019995. https://doi.org/10.1136/bmjopen-2017-019995

Banerjee, D., & Rao, T. S. (2022). The dark shadow of marital rape: Need to change the narrative. *Journal of Psychosexual Health, 4*(1), 11–13. https://doi.org/10.1177/26318318221083709

Bender, A. K., Koegler, E., Johnson, S. D., Murugan, V., & Wamser-Nanney, R. (2020). Guns and intimate partner violence among adolescents: A scoping review. *Journal of Family Violence, 36*, 605–617. https://doi.org/10.1007/s10896-20-00193x

Bennice, J., Resick, P., Mechanic, M., & Astin, M. (2019). The relative effects of intimate partner physical and sexual violence on posttraumatic stress disorder symptomatology. *Violence and Victims, 18*(1), 87–94. https://doi.org/10.1891/vivi.2003.18.1.87

Bernstein, P., Martin, J., Barton, J., Shields, L., Druzin, M., Scavone, B., Frost, J., Morton, C., Ruhl, C., Slager, J., Tzigas, E., Jaffer, S., & Menard, K. (2017). National partnership for maternal safety: Consensus bundle on severe hypertension, and the postpartum period. *Anesthesia and Analgesia, 125*(2), 540–547.

Bettinger-Lopez, C., & Bro, A. (2020). A double pandemic: Domestic violence in the age of COVID-19. *Gender-Based Violence, 3*. https://digitalcommons.wcl.american.edu/wlpviolence/3

Blaney, N., Randour, M., & Blink, C. (2021). Advances in understanding the link between pet abuse and intimate partner violence. In R. Geffner, J. W. White, L. K. Hamberger, A. Rosenbaum, V. Vaughn-Eden, & V. I. Vieth (Eds.), *Handbook of interpersonal violence and abuse across the lifespan* (pp. 2279–2300). Springer. https://doi.org/10.1007/978-3-319/89999-2_286

Bott, S., Guedes, A., Ruiz-Celis, A. P., & Mendoza, J. A. (2019). Intimate partner violence in the Americas: A systematic review and reanalysis of national prevalence estimates. *Pan American Journal of Public Health, 43*, e26. https://doi.org/10.26633/RPSP.2019.26

Boyce, S., Brouwer, K., Triplett, D., Servin, A., Magis-Rodriguez, C., & Silverman, J. (2018). Childhood experiences of sexual violence, pregnancy and marriage associated with child sex trafficking among female sex workers in two US-Mexican border cities. *American Journal of Public Health, 108*(8), 1049–1054. https://doi.org/10.2105/AJPH.2018.304455

Bozeman, J., Jones, R., & Loy, S. (2006). *Kennesaw.* Arcadia.

Campbell, A., Thompson, S., Harris, T., & Wiehe, S. (2018). Intimate partner violence and pet abuse: Responding law enforcement office observations and victim reports from the scene. *Journal of Interpersonal Violence, 36*(5–6), 2353–2372. https://doi.org/10.1177/0886260518759653

Chen, Y., Cheung, S., & Huang, C. (2020). Intimate partner violence during pregnancy: Effects of maternal depression and parenting on teen depressive symptoms. *Journal of Interpersonal Violence, 37*(9–10), 7034–7056.

Choi, J.-K., Kelley, M., Wang, D., & Kerby, H. (2021). Neighborhood environment and child health in immigrant families: Using nationally representative individual, family, and community datasets. *American Journal of Health Promotion, 35*(7), 948–956. https://doi.org/10.1177/08901171211012522

Collins, C., & Skarparis, K. (2020). The impact of human trafficking in relation to maternity care: A literature review. *Midwifery, 83*, 102645. https://doi.org/10.1016/j.midw.2020.102645. Epub2020 Jan 23.

Diaz, J., & Whitaker, R. (2013). Black mothers' perceptions about urban neighborhood safety and outdoor play for their preadolescent daughters. *Journal of Health Care for the Poor and Underserved, 24*(1), 206–219.

Ernewein, C., & Nieves, R. (2015). Human sex trafficking: Recognition, treatment, and referral of pediatric victims. *The Journal for Nurse Practitioners, 11*(8), 797–803.

Everytown for Gun Safety. (n.d.). Our mayors lead the way in advocating for gun safety in America. Everytown for Gun Safety, https://mayors.everytown.org/

Ficklin, E., Tehee, M., Killgore, R., Isaacs, D., Mack, S., & Ellington, T. (2021). Fighting for our sisters: Community advocacy and action for missing and murdered indigenous women and girls. *Journal of Social Issues, 78*(1), 53–78.

Fischer, C. (2008). Paradoxes of American individualism. *Sociological Forum, 23*(2), 363–365.

Geisbrecht, C. (2021). Intimate partner violence, animal maltreatment, and concern for animal safety: A survey of survivors who owned pets and livestock. *Violence Against Women, 28*, 2334. https://doi.org/10.1177/10778012211034215

Goodyear, A., Rodriguez, M., & Glik, D. (2020). The role of firearms in intimate partner violence: Policy and research considerations. *Journal of Public Health Policy, 41*, 185. https://doi.org/10.1057/s41271-019-00198-x

Gordon, M., Coverdale, J., Chervenak, F., & McCullough, L. (2022). Undue burdens created by the Texas abortion law for vulnerable women. *American Journal of Obstetrics and Gynecology, 226*(4), 529–534. https://doi.org/10.1016/j.ajog.2021.12.033

Gorodnichenko, Y., & Roland, G. (2021). Culture, institutions and democratization. *Public Choice, 187*(2), 165–195. https://doi.org/10.1007/s11127-020-00811-8

Healthy People 2030. (n.d.). U.S. Department of Health and Human Services, Office of Disease Prevention and Health Promotion. https://health.gov/healthypeople/objectives-and-data/social-determinants-health

Hill, N., & Herman-Stahl, M. (2002). Neighborhood safety and social involvement: Associations with parenting behaviors and depressive symptoms among African American and euro-American mothers. *Journal of Family Psychology, 16*(2), 209–219.

Hunt, B. (2021). Ain't no sunshine when she's gone: Missing and murdered indigenous women and girls in North Carolina. *North Carolina Medical Journal, 82*(6), 417–419.

Joseph, A. S. (2021). A modern trail of tears: The missing and murdered indigenous women crisis in US. *Journal of Forensic and Legal Medicine, 79*, 102–136.

Kaplan, D., Moore, J., Barron, C., & Goldberg, A. (2018). Domestic minor sex trafficking: Medical follow-up for victimized and high-risk youth. *Rhode Island Medical Journal.* www.rimed.org.

Kennedy, M. A., Arebalos, M., Ekroos, R., & Cimino, A. (2021). Sex trafficking red flags: Confirming presentation patterns and childhood adversity risk factors. *Nurse Leader, 19*(5), 516–520.

Koegler, E., Howland, W., Gibbons, P., Teti, M., & Stoklosa, H. (2020). "When her visa expired, the family refused to renew it," Intersection trafficking and domestic violence: Qualitative document analysis of C from a major Midwest city. *Journal of Interpersonal Violence, 37*, 133–159.

Laraia, B., Messer, L., Evenson, K., & Kaufman, J. (2007). Neighborhood factors associated with physical activity and adequacy of weight gain during pregnancy. *Journal of Urban Health, 84*, 793–806.

Le May, G. (2018). The cycles of violence against native women: An analysis of colonialism, historical legislation and the violence against women reauthorization act of 2013. *PSU McNair Scholars Online Journal, 12*(1), Article 1. https://doi.org/10.15760/mcnair.2018.1

Lucchesi, A., & Echo-Hawk, A. (2018). *Missing and murdered indigenous women and girls: A snapshot of data from 71 urban cities in the United States.* Urban India Health Institute. http://www.uihi.org/wp-content/uploads/2018/11/missing-and-murdered-indigenous-women-and-girls-report.pdf

MacDorman, M., Thoma, M., Deckercq, E., & Howell, E. (2021). Causes contributing to the excess of maternal mortality risk for women 35 and over United States, 2017–2018. *PLoS One, 16*(6), e0253920.

Malik, S., & Naeem, K. (2020). *Impact of Covid-19 on women: Health, livelihoods, and domestic violence.* Sustainable Development Policy Institute. http://hdl.handle.net/11540/11907

Mantegani, J. (2021). Slouching towards autonomy: Re-envisioning tribal jurisdiction, Native American autonomy, and violence against women in Indian country. *The Journal of Criminal Law and Criminology, 111*(1), 315–350.

Martin-Rogers, N., & Pendleton, V. (2020). *Missing and murdered indigenous women task force: A report to the Minnesota legislature* (pp. 1–154). Wilder Research. https://dps.mn.gov/divisions/ojp/Documents/missing-murdered-indigenous-women-task-force-report.pdf

Mayne, S. L., Pool, L. R., Grobman, W. A., & Kershaw, K. N. (2018). Associations of neighbourhood crime with adverse pregnancy outcomes among women in Chicago: Analysis of electronic health records from 2009 to 2013. *Journal of Epidemiology and Community Health, 72*(3), 230–236. https://doi.org/10.1136/jech-2017-209801

Middleton, J., Edwards, E., Roe-Sepowitz, D., Inman, E., Frey, L., & Gattis, M. (2022). Adverse childhood experiences (ACEs) and homelessness: A critical examination of the association between specific ACEs and sex trafficking among homeless youth in Kentuckiana. *Journal of Human Trafficking.* https://doi.org/10.1080/23322705.2021.20220061

Morton, R. (2016). Hitchhiking and missing and murdered indigenous women. *The Canadian Journal of Sociology, 41*(3), 299–326.

Murphy-Oikonen, J., Chambers, L., McQueen, K., Hiebert, A., & Miller, A. (2021). Sexual assault: Indigenous women's experiences of not being believed by the police. *Violence Against Women, 28*(5), 1237–1258. https://doi.org/10.1177/10778012211013903

Newman, B., & Hartman, T. (2017). Mass shootings and public support for gun control. *British Journal of Political Science, 49*(4), 1527–1553. https://doi.org/10.1017/S0007123417000333

Recknor, F., Gordon, M., Coverdale, J., Gardezi, M., & Nguyen, P. (2019). A descriptive study of United States-based human trafficking specialty clinics. *Psychiatric Quarterly, 91*, 1–10. https://doi.org/10.1007/s11126-019-09691-8

Reid, J., Baglivio, M., Piquero, A., Greenwald, M., & Epps, N. (2017). Human trafficking of minors and childhood adversity in Florida. *American Journal of Public Health, 107*(2), 306–311.

Schildkraut, J. (2019). A call to the media to change reporting practices for the coverage of mass shootings. *Washington University Journal of Law and Policy, 60*(1), 273–292. https://openscholarship.wustl.edu/law_journal_law_policy/vol60/iss1/16

Shah, L., Varma, B., Nasir, K., Walsh, M., Blumenthal, R., Mehta, L., & Sharma, G. (2021). Reducing disparities in adverse pregnancy outcomes in the United States. *American Heart Journal, 242*, 92–102.

Shannon, M., Clougherty, J., McCarthy, C., Elovitz, M., Tiako, M., Melly, S., & Burris, H. (2020). Neighborhood violent crime and perceived stress in pregnancy. *International Journal of Environmental Research, 17*(15), 5585.

Sharma, R., Pooyak, S., Jongbloed, K., Zamar, D., Pearce, M., Mazzuca, A., Schecter, M., & Spittal, P. (2021). The Cedar Project: Historical, structural, and interpersonal determinants of involvement in survival sex work over time among indigenous women who have used drugs in two Canadian cities. *International Journal of Drug Policy, 87*, 103012. https://doi.org/10.2196/16783

Shields, L., Wiesner, S., Fulton, J., & Pelletreau, B. (2015). Comprehensive maternal hemorrhage protocols reduce the use of blood products and improve patient safety. *American Journal of Obstetrics and Gynecology, 212*(3), 272–280.

Simpson, J. (2021). Growing burdens on abortion rights: An individual freedom during Covid-19 and changing judicial interpretation. *Mitchell Hamline Law Journal of Public Policy and Practice, 42*(2), Article 3. https://open.mitchellhamline.edu/policypractice/vol42/iss2/3

Sojourner Center. (2022). Emergency support services: Pet companion shelter. para 1. https://www.sojournercenter.org/pet-companion-shelter/

Sorenson, S., & Schut, R. (2018). Non-fatal gun use in intimate partner violence: A systematic review of the literature. *Trauma, Violence, and Abuse, 19*(4), 431–442.

Spitzer, R. J. (2020). *The politics of gun control*. Routledge.

Stanhope, K. K., Adeyemi, D. I., Li, T., Johnson, T., & Boulet, S. L. (2021). The relationship between the neighborhood built and social environment and hypertensive disorders of pregnancy: A scoping review. *Annals of Epidemiology, 64*, 67–75. https://doi.org/10.1016/j.annepidem.2021.09.005

Stevenson, R., Fitzgerald, A., & Barrett, B. (2017). Keeping pets safe in the context of intimate partner violence: Insights from domestic violence shelter staff in Canada. *Affilia, 33*(2), 236–252. https://doi.org/10.1177/0886109917747613

Stoklosa, H., Alhajii, L., Finch, L., Williams, S., Sfakianaki, A., Duhely, L., & Potter, J. (2022). Because the resources aren't there, then we fail. We fail as a society: A qualitative analysis of human trafficking provider perceptions of child welfare involvement among trafficked mothers. *Maternal and Child Health Journal, 26*, 623–631.

Turner, M. (2019). Maternal sepsis is an evolving challenge. *Gynecology and Obstetrics, 146*(1), 39–42. https://doi.org/10.1002/ijgo.12833

Twis, M., Gillespie, L., & Geenwood, D. (2020). An analysis of romantic partner dynamics in domestic minor sex trafficking files. *Journal of Interpersonal Violence, 37*, 394–418.

United States Department of Justice. (2022). Project safe neighborhood: *Topics*. https://www.justice.gov/topics

Waterman, A. (1981). Individualism and interdependence. *American Psychologist, 36*(7), 762–773.

White House. (2022). The National Action Plan to combat Human Trafficking (pp. 1–66). https://www.whitehouse.gov/wp-content/uploads/2021/12/National-Action-Plan-to-Combat-Human-Trafficking.pdf

Xie, Y., & Lou, Z. (2022). Effective organization management in multinational corporations: In the context of collectivism and individualism. *Advances in Social Science, Education, Humanities Research, 638*, 712–717.

Yakubovich, A. R., Stöckl, H., Murray, J., Melendez-Torres, G. J., Steinert, J. I., Glavin, C., & Humphreys, D. K. (2018). Risk and protective factors for intimate partner violence against women: Systematic review and meta-analyses of prospective-longitudinal studies. *American Journal of Public Health, 108*(7), e1–e11. https://doi.org/10.2105/AJPH.2018.304428

Chapter 14
Substance Use and Maternal Health

Linda R. McDaniel

14.1 Substance Use and Maternal Health Outcomes

Substance use during pregnancy is known to have potentially adverse effects on maternal and fetal outcomes. Substance use and opioid use disorders in the USA have progressively worsened over the decades, despite local, state, and federal initiatives. Substance use in pregnancy is a growing public health concern. The National Survey on Drug Use and Health (2011–2012) reported that on average, 5.9% of pregnant individuals aged 15–44 use illicit drugs. The rate of substance use varies by age group; those 15–17 years had the highest rate (18.3%), ages 18–25 (9.0%), and ages 26–44 (3.4%). Another area of growing concern is pregnancy-associated mortality involving opioids (American Society of Addiction Medicine, 2017; Gemmill et al., 2019). From 2010 to 2019, a study which evaluated pregnancy-associated deaths that resulted from drug overdose, suicide, and homicide found that 11.4% of the 11,782 death certificates reviewed were related to drugs. Their findings indicate that pregnancy-associated deaths due to drug use have overwhelmingly increased by 190% during this time period (Margerison et al., 2022).

Issues surrounding substance use disorders are complex. Substance-using mothers may find it very difficult to discontinue. Factors that influence maternal substance use disorders may be biological, behavioral, environmental, and/or psychological trauma, including physical and sexual abuse. These factors contribute to adverse social determinants of health (SDoH) including but not limited to access to healthcare, stigmatism, discrimination, socioeconomic instability, inadequate housing, and pressures to comply with societal rules and expectations despite the challenges they face while raising their families and trying to be *good* mothers

L. R. McDaniel (✉)
Healthcare Provider, WellStar Medical Group Cobb Gynecologists, Austell, GA, USA

© The Author(s), under exclusive license to Springer Nature Switzerland AG 2023
B. A. Anderson, L. R. Roberts (eds.), *Maternal Health and American Cultural Values*,
Global Maternal and Child Health, https://doi.org/10.1007/978-3-031-23969-4_14

(Goldstein et al., 2021; Gemmill et al., 2019; Substance Abuse and Mental Health Services Administration, 2021; Van Scoyoc et al., 2017; Wang et al., 2020).

14.2   The Influence of Self-Reliance

Self-reliance is a key American cultural value that views the individual as an autonomous, self-sufficient person who is expected to take responsibility, without undue dependence upon others. Self-reliance is also known as "bootstrapping." Individuals should rely upon themselves to get their lives in order. The American culture views substance use during pregnancy in a negative light, considering these women to be weak, lacking in self-reliance, and placing blame on the individuals for having this problem (Weber et al., 2021; Van Scoyoc et al., 2017). Pregnancy is socially viewed as a time when women should disregard their personal challenges and stop using any substances that could harm the unborn child. In fact, many pregnant women *do* stop using substances harmful to themselves or the unborn child. There are some, however, who are unable to stop using or resume use during the postpartum period. Resuming drug use is viewed as a lack of self-control and self-reliance and this behavior is strongly condemned. This high sense of disapproval may be expressed overtly or experienced implicitly. It results in stigmatization, a form of discrimination, negatively impacting the mothers' ability to receive proper care and treatment. When these individuals present for prenatal care and those who muster the courage to disclose their substance use history, they are often misunderstood by those caring for them. The message is that it is their fault. Thus, they are then lectured about what can happen to them and/or their unborn child if they continue to use drugs during pregnancy. They are admonished to "stop" using. These messages do not foster kindness, support, encouragement, and empowerment needed for self-care during childbearing.

14.3   Complexities of Receiving Prenatal Care

Substance use during pregnancy is often intertwined with mental health disorders (American Society of Addiction Medicine, 2017; Arnaudo et al., 2017; Haffajee et al., 2021). Many mothers with substance use disorder delay prenatal care and treatment because of stigmatization, discrimination, and punitive consequences. Often mothers with substance abuse disorders may wait to establish care into the second or third trimester, attend less than 5 prenatal visits, or drop in at their local hospital as needed. They face repetitive judgmental comments and dismissive attitudes when they bring up a concern and they often feel a loss of autonomy and self-reliance. The situation is further compounded by the inability to meet cultural expectations to be self-reliant in discontinuing substance use, adding guilt and shame, resulting in avoidance or delay in seeking prenatal care (Amnesty International, 2017; Nichols et al., 2021; Wang et al., 2020).

14.3.1 Stigmatization and Discrimination

In general, individuals with a substance use disorder are often misunderstood, facing stigma and discrimination in all aspects of life. This stigma is magnified for pregnant women who use substances. When talking about substance use, it is generally referred to as substance *abuse*. This disease-oriented terminology is enshrined by its frequent use in laws, the media, healthcare settings, and society at large, further alienating these individuals (Atayde et al., 2021; Bessette et al., 2022; Muncan et al., 2020). Social labels used to describe substance-using individuals include junkie, addict, crackhead, user, alcoholic, drunk, former addict, and reformed addict. These labels indicate that the individual *is* the problem rather than *has* a problem (National Institute on Drug Abuse, 2021a). This language produces a skewed lens through which the individual is perceived and treated. This terminology lends to the perception that individuals who use substances are a threat to society and willfully engage in these activities, warranting punitive measures (Atayde et al., 2021; Escañuela Sánchez et al., 2022; Krans et al., 2019; Muncan et al., 2020; National Institute on Drug Abuse, 2021a, b; Weber et al., 2021).

Due to gender and social norms, women with substance use disorders seem to experience stigma more often than males. Mothers with substance use disorders are labeled as irresponsible, negligent, selfish, and violating the moral code of parenthood. Stigma perpetuates the assault, adding to their emotional scars, further impacting mental health, and a sense of a disempowerment (Renbarger et al., 2020). The stigma and negative stereotyping are internalized; women begin to believe these messages exacerbating poor self-image (Atayde et al., 2021; Escañuela Sánchez et al., 2022; Weber et al., 2021). Feelings of shame, guilt, fear, depression, and anxiety can negatively influence willingness to seek and receive prenatal, primary, or mental healthcare (American Psychiatric Association, 2016; Atayde et al., 2021; Escañuela Sánchez et al., 2022; Faherty et al., 2019; Goldstein et al., 2021; Nichols et al., 2021; Paris et al., 2020; Syvertsen et al., 2021; Toquinto et al., 2020).

14.3.2 Legal Ramifications

The majority of professional and federal organizations have found that current federal and state punitive statutes can be detrimental to maternal and fetal well-being (Faherty et al., 2019; Ecker et al., 2019). Some state legislatures have developed punitive legislation to address the growing pregnancy-associated substance use problem, thus criminally prosecuting and incarcerating mothers (Angelotta & Appelbaum, 2017; Escañuela Sánchez et al., 2022; Daniel, 2019; Goldstein et al.,

2021; Guttmacher Institute, 2021; Haffajee et al., 2021; Jarlenski et al., 2017; Van Scoyoc et al., 2017). According to McVay (2021), at the end of 2018, 26% and 24% of female *state* prisoners were serving time for drug-related offenses and property-related offenses respectively. In 2019, based upon Department of Justice data, 6500 (59%) female *federal* prisoners were serving time for drug-related offenses. Many of these prisoners were pregnant or parenting. Recent findings indicate that around 50% of all incarcerated with non-affective psychosis or documented depression are substance-abusing (Baranyi et al., 2022).

The Child Abuse Prevention and Treatment Act (CAPTA) is a federal law that allows state governments to receive federal grants that focus on child abuse and neglect prevention. In order for state governments to receive these funds, they must have mandatory reporting policies. Healthcare providers involved in the care of mothers who use substances during pregnancy, or to infants born who are affected by perinatal drug exposure, are required to contact local child protective services agencies (Falletta et al., 2018; Haffajee et al., 2021; Jarlenski et al., 2017; Krans et al., 2019). There are, however, variations in state laws. In nine states, healthcare providers potentially face a misdemeanor charge if they fail to report known occurrences of mothers who use substances during pregnancy. According to the statutes in some states, healthcare providers can file a report if they think a woman is using substances during pregnancy even without concrete evidence. Some state laws inflict punitive actions if mothers with substance use disorders do not initiate or complete treatment (Jarlenski et al., 2017). This poses a significant quandary of trust for both parties and it further perpetuates discrimination against pregnant and parenting mothers.

The National Center on Substance Abuse and Child Welfare (2019) reports that from 2000 to 2019, the prevalence of substance abuse as a condition for child removal increased from 18.5% to 38.9%. Child protective reporting is state mandated; however, bias can play a role in reporting as there are no standardized hospital reporting protocols (Goldstein et al., 2021; Harp & Oser, 2018; Rebbe et al., 2019). According to the United States Department of Health and Human Services [USDHHS] Children's Bureau (2020), there are 26 states and the District of Columbia that have laws and policies regarding mandatory reporting of perinatal substance exposure. However, only 23 states and the District of Columbia provide definitions of what constitutes perinatal substance abuse. Lack of reporting leads to discrepancies in data due to lack of knowledge by health providers, concerns about interrupting the maternal-infant dyad, mistrust of or negative experience with Child Protective Services (CPS), or having to testify in a CPS case. Racial bias has been shown to be significant in the reporting process. Putnum-Hornstein et al. (2016) found in their research of Black, Hispanic, and White infants born within the California 2006 birth cohort that White mothers had more occurrences of perinatal substance use but Black and Hispanic substance-exposed infants were more frequently reported to CPS than White infants. Rebbe et al. (2019) found that the

Washington State minimizes the number of infants reported to CPS during the neonatal period to avoid disruption of the mother-infant. In Rhode Island, CPS investigation only occurs if there is allegation of newborn or child abuse/neglect occurring in the home (USDHHS, 2020).

The threat or actual prosecution of criminalization can positively or negatively impact the mother's response and her subsequent health outcomes. For some mothers, if not properly treated for drug use, there is a high rate of relapse. The threat of criminalization does *not* motivate self-reliance to seek permanent cessation. For others, potential criminalization may be the turning point that inspires self-reliant treatment-seeking behavior and permanent refrain from substances (Amnesty International, 2017; Escañuela Sánchez et al., 2022; Van Scoyoc et al., 2017).

14.4 Adverse Social Determinants of Health

Mothers with substance use disorders encounter many challenges that affect their livelihoods and ability to care for themselves. Structural and societal factors such as the ability to access healthcare, poverty, and inadequate insurance, unstable housing, and limited transportation are key SDoH that affect maternal health outcomes (Wang et al., 2020). Yet, supportive social and community factors can play a pivotal role in mitigating these adverse SDoH and prevent poor maternal health outcomes (Creary-Perry et al., 2021; Escañuela Sánchez et al., 2022; Gadson et al., 2017; Meyer et al., 2016; Kramlich et al., 2018).

14.4.1 Low Socioeconomic Status

A mother's socioeconomic status is key to meeting basic needs. Mothers with substance use disorders tend to be of lower socioeconomic status, increasing vulnerability to adverse maternal outcomes related to poverty and lack of financial stability for themselves and their children. When faced with challenges in meeting basic needs (e.g., food, water, housing, etc.) versus paying for insurance, co-pays, or deductibles, American mothers sacrifice healthcare to ensure that basic necessities are met. Poverty and low socioeconomic status play a significant role in meeting healthcare needs (Gadson et al., 2017; Henry et al., 2021). Mothers of lower socioeconomic status often have poor prenatal utilization, with late initiation of care (second or third trimester), limited or inconsistent prenatal care, increasing the risk of poor maternal health outcomes (Gadson et al., 2017; Kramlich et al., 2018).

14.4.2   Inadequate Insurance Coverage

The ability to secure services is a key factor in overall health. In the USA, Medicaid is the primary insurance provider for two-thirds of mothers ages 19 to 49. American women with substance use disorders typically have no insurance, but may have Medicaid or Medicare (Bigby et al., 2020; Haffajee et al., 2021). They often enter care late due to barriers in obtaining health insurance. Access to care can be further complicated for mothers residing in healthcare shortage areas where prenatal care providers and substance use treatment centers are limited (Bigby et al., 2020; Meyer et al., 2016; Patrick et al., 2020). An additional challenge is that Medicaid coverage expires three months after childbirth. These issues are compounded for substance-abusing mothers who lack coverage and access to addiction treatment. However, the Affordable Care Act has improved this situation for non-insured substance-abusing mothers.

14.4.3   Unstable Housing and Limited Transportation

Homelessness and isolation contribute to maternal morbidity and mortality. In particular, homeless substance-abusing mothers are more likely to have increased episodes of malnutrition and decreased weight gain resulting in either growth restricted or small for gestational age infants. Also, I (LMcD) have found that homeless individuals may not provide full disclosure of living conditions at the time of hospital discharge where these individuals continue to face resource issues to properly feed and care for themselves and the newborn. Housing instability can consist of various forms of homelessness: episodic, transitional, chronic, and rural. These kinds of homelessness are often in tandem with lack of access to transportation. Homeless mothers are likely to live in emergency shelters (United States Department of Housing and Urban Development, 2020). Compounding the issue is that most transitional housing programs do not admit substance-abusing mothers forcing them back to the streets. When faced with homelessness, many American mothers seek to be self-reliant, establishing networks and seeking resources to improve their housing dilemma (Knight, 2017; Frazer et al., 2019). These networks may be kinship, social services, faith-based organizations, or "fictive" kinship among non-blood-related persons. Any of these sources can foster empowerment and build self-reliance. Substance-abusing mothers often lack the coping and navigation skills to avoid isolation, break damaging relationships, and develop social networks (Escañuela Sánchez et al., 2022; Knight, 2017). Asta et al. (2021) report that substance use during pregnancy can have the ability to change (intrinsic) and break harmful social relationships (extrinsic).

14.4.4 Community Response to Substance-Abusing Mothers

The response of the community may be a double-edged sword for pregnant and parenting mothers with substance use disorders. The community has the power to exacerbate feelings of guilt and foster the environment for poor maternal outcomes. Social disapproval equated with being a "bad mother," perpetuates negative feelings as these mothers navigate the path to cessation (Escañuela Sánchez et al., 2022; Toquinto et al., 2020; Nichols et al., 2021). Conversely, when drug-free social networks are readily available, offer encouragement toward responsible motherhood, and promote self-reliance, the substance-abusing mother has a chance to move toward positive health behavior change (Ades et al., 2018; American Psychiatric Association, 2016; Asta et al., 2021).

14.5   The Means to Overcome

There is a myth that mothers are unmotivated to be drug-free and are unconcerned about the effects on their previously born or unborn children. This myth fosters stigma, discrimination, and criminalization. Many substance-abusing mothers avoid initiating care because they are afraid of the negative consequences of disclosure or discovery. Prior to or instead of seeking healthcare services, they may try to help themselves by limiting access to drugs, weaning, changing, or stopping abruptly (*cold turkey*). They may seek to be self-reliant by seeking information, eating a healthy diet, exercising, getting adequate sleep, and taking prenatal vitamins (Escañuela Sánchez et al., 2022; Goldstein et al., 2021; Goodman et al., 2020; Frazer et al., 2019; Meyer et al., 2016; Van Scoyoc et al., 2017). When they do enter care, they are criticized for avoiding care or waiting too long. This social response is punishing to the mother who finally makes a move toward trust.

Instead, they need to be embraced and praised for the courage to face the issue positively. The mantle of motherhood, the self-image of oneself as a mother, may, in itself, be a significant motivator to reduce drug use and to achieve long-term abstinence (Cleveland et al., 2016; Goodman et al., 2020; Nichols et al., 2021). I have found that being the light of hope for these individuals is key when caring for them during pregnancy. Substance-using mothers have told me that treating them as a person and not shaming them has given them the strength to keep coming to their appointments, with the courage to proceed with birth and motherhood despite their current circumstances.

In describing processes that promote successful remission among substance-abusing mothers, Moos (2007) reports that treatment requires individual motivation, established goals, a positive social network, effective coping mechanisms, and development of self-efficacy. The following is a composite exemplar of three substance-abusing mothers who faced many adverse SDoH but who learned the skills of motherhood and built networks to be clean, sober, and self-reliant.

> **Box 14.1 Three Stories of Drug-Using Mothers (Linda McDaniel, DNP, CNM, June 10, 2022)**
>
> Alice was a victim of intimate partner violence, depression, and substance use. She recounts how most healthcare personnel she encountered during her childbearing experiences made her feel worse. One pivotal encounter with a providers took the time to make it safe to tell her story. Alice says she felt "free" after telling her story and that provider gave her hope and encouragement that she could change her life. That provider was instrumental in getting her into a program for treatment and counseling.
>
> Briana reports that pregnancy was the turning point in stopping the use of substances. She said, "It became real for me and I wanted to give my children every chance possible." She says pregnancy "saved me".
>
> Cathy reports using substances during her first pregnancy and had a pre-term delivery at 33 weeks. Her infant had multiple complications and died. She reports that the death of child sent her into a tailspin of depression, binge drug use and attempted suicide. In the ER with this suicide attempt, she found out she was pregnant again. This was the pivotal point when she could make amends to her first child. She sought treatment and went on to have three healthy children.

14.6   Summary

Most substance-abusing mothers are concerned about the impact of drug use upon their children and themselves. They aspire to be good mothers. In a supportive, non-discriminating environment that embraces and builds upon the American cultural value of self-reliance, they can be encouraged to seek and maintain treatment (Cleveland et al., 2016; Goodman et al., 2020).

However, healthcare and legislative reform is essential in promoting policies and programs that decriminalize the mother, provide a supportive milieu, and encourage health-seeking behaviors.

References

Ades, V., Goddard, B., Pearson Ayala, S., Chemouni Bach, S., & Wu, S. X. (2018, June 1). ACOG Committee Opinion No. 729: Importance of social determinants of health and cultural awareness in the delivery of reproductive health care. *Obstetrics and Gynecology, 131*(6), 1162–1163. https://doi.org/10.1097/aog.0000000000002660

American Psychiatric Association. (2016). *American psychiatric association position statement: Assuring the appropriate care of pregnant and newly-delivered women with substance use disorders.* American Psychiatric Association.

American Society of Addiction Medicine. (2017). Public policy statement on substance use, misuse, and use disorders during and following pregnancy, with an emphasis on opioids. *American*

Society of Addiction Medicine. https://www.asam.org/advocacy/public-policy-statements/details/public-policy-statements/2021/08/09/substance-use-misuse-and-use-disorders-during-and-following-pregnancy-with-an-emphasis-on-opioids

Amnesty International. (2017). USA: Criminalizing pregnancy: Policing pregnant women who use drugs in the USA. *Amnesty International.* https://www.amnestyusa.org/reports/criminalizing-pregnancy-policing-pregnant-women-use-drugs-usa/

Angelotta, C., & Appelbaum, P. S. (2017). Criminal charges for child harm from substance use in pregnancy. *Journal of the American Academy of Psychiatry and the Law, 45*(2), 193–203.

Arnaudo, C. L., Andraka-Christou, B., & Allgood, K. (2017). Psychiatric co-morbidities in pregnant women with opioid use disorders: Prevalence, impact, and implications for treatment. *Current Addiction Reports, 4*(1), 1–13. https://doi.org/10.1007/s40429-017-0132-4

Asta, D., Davis, A., Krishnamurti, T., Klocke, L., Abdullah, W., & Krans, E. E. (2021). The influence of social relationships on substance use behaviors among pregnant women with opioid use disorder. *Drug and Alcohol Dependence, 222*, 108665. https://doi.org/10.1016/j.drugalcdep.2021.108665

Atayde, A. M. P., Hauc, S. C., Bessette, L. G., Danckers, H., & Saitz, R. (2021). Changing the narrative: A call to end stigmatizing terminology related to substance use disorders. *Addiction Research & Theory, 29*(5), 359–362. https://doi.org/10.1080/16066359.2021.1875215

Baranyi, G., Fazel, S., Delhey Langerfeldt, S., & Mundt, A. (2022). The prevalence of comorbid serious mental illnesses and substance use disorders in prison populations: A systematic review and meta-analysis. *The Lancet, 7*, e557–e568. www.thelancet.com/public-health open access

Bessette, L. G., Hauc, S. C., Danckers, H., Atayde, A., & Saitz, R. (2022). The associated press stylebook changes and the use of addiction-related stigmatizing terms in news media. *Substance Abuse, 43*(1), 127–130. https://pubmed.ncbi.nlm.nih.gov/32348190/. https://doi.org/10.1080/08897077.2020.1748167

Bigby, J., Anthony, J., Hsu, R., Fiorentini, C., & Rosenbach, M. (2020). Recommendations for maternal health and infant health quality improvement in Medicaid and the children's health insurance program. *Medicaid & CHIP Maternal and Infant Health Quality Improvement.* https://www.medicaid.gov/medicaid/quality-of-care/downloads/mih-expert-workgroup-recommendations.pdf

Cleveland, L. M., Bonugli, R. J., & McGlothen, K. S. (2016). The mothering experiences of women with substance use disorders. *Advances in Nursing Science, 39*(2), 119–129. https://doi.org/10.1097/ANS.0000000000000118

Creary-Perry, J., Correa-de-Araujo, R., Lewis Johnson, T., McLemore, M. R., Neilson, E., & Wallace, M. (2021). Social and structural determinants of health inequities in maternal health. *Journal of Women's Health, 30*(2), 230–235. https://doi.org/10.1089/jwh.2020.8882

Daniel, R. (2019). Prisons neglect pregnant women in their healthcare policies. *Prison Policy Initiative.* https://www.prison policy.org/blog/2019/12/05/pregnancy/

Ecker, J., Abuhamad, A., Hill, W., Bailit, J., Bateman, B. T., Berghella, V., Blake-Lamb, T., Guille, C., Landau, R., Minkoff, H., Prabhu, M., Rosenthal, E., Terplan, M., Wright, T. E., & Yonkers, K. A. (2019). Substance use disorders in pregnancy: Clinical, ethical, and research imperatives of the opioid epidemic: A report of a joint workshop of the Society for Maternal-Fetal Medicine, American College of Obstetricians and Gynecologists, and American Society of Addiction Medicine. *American Journal of Obstetrics and Gynecology, 221*(1), B5–B28. https://doi.org/10.1016/j.ajog.2019.03.022

Escañuela Sánchez, T., Matvienko-Sikar, K., Linehan, L., O'Donoghue, K., Byrne, M., & Meaney, S. (2022). Facilitators and barriers to substance-free pregnancies in high-income countries: A meta-synthesis of qualitative research. *Women and Birth: Journal of the Australian College of Midwives, 35*(2), e99–e110. https://doi.org/10.1016/j.wombi.2021.04.010

Faherty, L. J., Kranz, A. M., Russell-Fritch, J., Patrick, S. W., Cantor, J., & Stein, B. D. (2019). Association of punitive and reporting state policies related to substance use in pregnancy with rates of neonatal abstinence syndrome. *JAMA Network Open, 2*(11), e1914078. https://doi.org/10.1001/jamanetworkopen.2019.14078

Falletta, L., Hamilton, K., Fischbein, R., Aultman, J., Kinney, B., & Kenne, D. (2018). Perceptions of child protective services among pregnant or recently pregnant, opioid-using women in substance abuse treatment. *Child Abuse & Neglect, 79*, 125–135. https://doi.org/10.1016/j. drugalcdep.2019.107652

Frazer, Z., McConnell, K., & Jansson, L. M. (2019). Treatment for substance use disorders in pregnant women: Motivators and barriers. *Drug and Alcohol Dependence, 205*, 107652. https://doi. org/10.1016/j.drugalcdep.2019.107652

Gadson, A., Akpovi, E., & Mehta, P. K. (2017). Exploring the social determinants of racial/ethnic disparities in prenatal care utilization and maternal outcome. *Seminars in Perinatology, 41*(5), 308–317. https://doi.org/10.1053/j.semperi.2017.04.008

Gemmill, A., Kiang, M. V., & Alexander, M. J. (2019). Trends in pregnancy-associated mortality involving opioids in the United States, 2007-2016. *American Journal of Obstetrics and Gynecology, 220*(1), 115–116. https://doi.org/10.1016/j.ajog.2018.09.028

Goldstein, E., Nervik, K., Hagen, S., Hilliard, F., Turnquiat, A., Bakhireva, L., McDonald, R., Ossorio, P., Lo, J., & Zgierska, A. (2021, September–October). A socioecological framework for engaging substance-using pregnant persons in longitudinal research: Multi-stakeholder perspectives. *Neurotoxicology and Teratology, 87*, 106997. https://doi.org/10.1016/j. ntt.2021.106997

Goodman, D. J., Saunders, E. C., & Wolff, K. B. (2020). In their own words: A qualitative study of factors promoting resilience and recovery among postpartum women with opioid use disorders. *BMC Pregnancy and Childbirth, 20*(1), 178. https://doi.org/10.1186/s12884-020-02872-5

Guttmacher Institute. (2021). Substance use during pregnancy. *Guttmacher Institute*. https://www. guttmacher.org/state-policy/explore/substance-use-during-pregnancy

Haffajee, R. L., Faherty, L. J., & Zivin, K. (2021). Pregnant women with substance use disorders—The harm associated with punitive approaches. *The New England Journal of Medicine, 384*(25), 2364–2367. https://doi.org/10.1097/01.aoa.0000816752.92932.36

Harp, K. L. H., & Oser, C. B. (2018). A longitudinal analysis of the impact of child custody loss on drug use and crime among a sample of African American mothers. *Child Abuse & Neglect, 77*, 1–12. https://doi.org/10.1016/j.chiabu.2017.12.017

Henry, M. C., Sanjuan, P. M., Stone, L. C., Cairo, G. F., Lohr-Valdez, A., & Leeman, L. M. (2021). Alcohol and other substance use disorder recovery during pregnancy among patients with post-traumatic stress disorder symptoms: A qualitative study. *Drug and Alcohol Dependence, 1*, 100013. https://doi.org/10.1016/j.dadr.2021.100013

Jarlenski, M., Hogan, C., Bogen, D. L., Chang, J. C., Bodnar, L. M., & Van Nostrand, E. (2017). Characterization of U.S. state laws requiring health care provider reporting of perinatal substance use. *Women's Health Issues, 27*(3), 264–270. https://doi.org/10.1016/j.whi.2016.12.008

Knight, C. (2017). Group work with homeless mothers: Promoting resilience through mutual aid. *Social Work, 62*(3), 235–242. https://doi.org/10.1093/sw/swx022

Kramlich, D., Kronk, R., Marcellus, L., Colbert, A., & Jakub, K. (2018). Rural postpartum women with substance use disorders. *Qualitative Health Research, 28*(9), 1449–1461. https://doi. org/10.1177/1049732318765720

Krans, E. E., Campopiano, M., Cleveland, L. M., Goodman, D., Kilday, D., Kendig, S., Leffert, L. R., Main, E. K., Mitchell, K. T., O'Gurek, D. T., D'Oria, R., McDaniel, D., & Terplan, M. (2019). National partnership for maternal safety: Consensus bundle on obstetric care for women with opioid use disorder. *Obstetrics and Gynecology, 134*(2), 365–375. https://doi. org/10.1097/AOG.0000000000003381

Margerison, C. E., Roberts, M. H., Gemmill, A., & Goldman-Mellor, S. (2022). Pregnancy-associated deaths due to drugs, suicide, and homicide in the United States, 2010–2019. *Obstetrics & Gynecology, 139*(2), 172–180. https://doi.org/10.1097/AOG.0000000000004649

McVay, D. (2021). Drugs and the prison, jail, probation, and parole systems. *Drug Policy Facts*. https://www.drugpolicyfacts.org/chapter/drug_prison

Meyer, E., Hennink, M., Rochat, R., Julian, Z., Pinto, M., Zertuche, A. D., Spelke, B., Dott, A., & Cota, P. (2016). Working towards safe motherhood: Delays and barriers to prenatal care for women in rural and peri-urban areas of Georgia. *Maternal and Child Health Journal, 20*(7), 1358–1365. https://doi.org/10.1007/s10995-016-1997-x

Moos, R. H. (2007). Theory-based processes that promote the remission of substance use disorders. *Clinical Psychology Review, 27*(5), 537–551. https://doi.org/10.1016/j.cpr.2006.12.006

Muncan, B., Walters, S. M., Ezell, J., & Ompad, D. C. (2020). "They look at us like junkies": Influences of drug use stigma on the healthcare engagement of people who inject drugs in New York City. *Harm Reduction Journal, 17*(1), 53. https://doi.org/10.1186/s12954-020-00399-8

National Center on Substance Abuse and Child Welfare. (2019). Child welfare and alcohol and drug use statistics. *National Center on Substance Abuse and Child Welfare.* https://ncsacw.acf.hhs.gov/research/child-welfare-and-treatment-statistics.aspx

National Institute on Drug Abuse. (2021a). Words matter—Terms to use and avoid when talking about addiction. *National Institute on Drug Abuse.* https://nida.nih.gov/nidamed-medical-health-professionals/health-professions-education/words-matter-terms-to-use-avoid-when-talking-about-addiction

National Institute on Drug Abuse. (2021b). Your words matter – Language showing compassion and care for women, infants, families, and communities impacted by substance use disorder. *National Institute on Drug Abuse.* https://nida.nih.gov/nidamed-medical-health-professionals/health-professions-education/words-matter-language-showing-compassion-care-women-infants-families-communities-impacted-substance-use-disorder

Nichols, T. R., Welborn, A., Gringle, M. R., & Lee, A. (2021). Social stigma and perinatal substance use services: Recognizing the power of the good mother ideal. *Contemporary Drug Problems, 48*(1), 19–37. https://doi.org/10.1177/0091450920969200

Paris, R., Herriott, A. L., Maru, M., Hacking, S. E., & Sommer, A. R. (2020). Secrecy versus disclosure: Women with substance use disorders share experiences in help seeking during pregnancy. *Maternal and Child Health Journal, 24*(11), 1396–1403. https://doi.org/10.1007/s10995-020-03006-1

Patrick, S. W., Richards, M. R., Dupont, W. D., McNeer, E., Buntin, M. B., Martin, P. R., Davis, M. M., Davis, C. S., Hartmann, K. E., Leech, A. A., Lovell, K. S., Stein, B. D., & Cooper, W. O. (2020). Association of pregnancy and insurance status with treatment access for opioid use disorder. *JAMA Network Open, 3*(8), e2013456. https://doi.org/10.1001/jamanetworkopen.2020.13456

Putnum-Hornstein, E., Prindle, J. J., & Leventhal, J. M. (2016). Prenatal substance exposure and reporting of child maltreatment by race and ethnicity. *Pediatrics, 138*(3), 1. https://doi.org/10.1542/peds.2016-1273

Rebbe, R., Mienko, J. A., Brown, E., & Rowhani-Rahbar, A. (2019). Hospital variation in child protection reports of substance exposed infants. *The Journal of Pediatrics, 208*, 141. https://doi.org/10.1016/j.jpeds.2018.12.065

Renbarger, K. M., Shieh, C., Moorman, M., Latham-Mintus, K., & Draucker, C. (2020). Health care encounters of pregnant and postpartum women with substance use disorders. *Western Journal of Nursing Research, 42*(8), 612–628. https://doi.org/10.1177/0193945919893372

Substance Abuse and Mental Health Services Administration. (2021). Addressing the specific needs of women for treatment of substance use disorders. *Publication No. PEP20-06-04-002.* https://store.samhsa.gov/sites/default/files/SAMHSA_Digital_Download/PEP20-06-04-002.pdf

Syvertsen, J. L., Toneff, H., Howard, H., Spadola, C., Madden, D., & Clapp, J. (2021). Conceptualizing stigma in contexts of pregnancy and opioid misuse: A qualitative study with women and healthcare providers in Ohio. *Drug and Alcohol Dependence, 222*, 108677. https://doi.org/10.1016/j.drugalcdep.2021.108677

Toquinto, S. M., Berglas, N. F., McLemore, M. R., Delgado, A., & Roberts, S. C. M. (2020). Pregnant women's acceptability of alcohol, tobacco, and drug use screening and willingness to disclose use in prenatal care. *Women's Health Issues, 30*(5), 345–352. https://doi.org/10.1016/j.whi.2020.05.004

United States Department of Health and Human Services, Children's Bureau. (2020). Child welfare information gateway. Parental drug use as child abuse. https://www.childwelfare.gov/pubPDFs/parentailsubstanceuse.pdf

United States Department of Housing and Urban Development. (2020). Continuum of care homeless populations and subpopulations. *HUD Exchange*. https://www.hudexchange.info/programs/coc/coc-homeless-populations-and-subpopulations-reports/

Van Scoyoc, A., Harrison, J., & Fisher, P. (2017). Beliefs and behaviors of pregnant women with addictions awaiting treatment initiation. *Child and Adolescent Social Work, 3*(1), 65–79. https://doi.org/10.1007/s10560-016-0474-0

Wang, E., Glazer, K. B., Howell, E. A., & Janevic, T. M. (2020). Social determinants of pregnancy-related mortality and morbidity in the United States: A systematic review. *Obstetrics and Gynecology, 135*(4), 896–915. https://doi.org/10.1097/AOG.0000000000003762

Weber, A., Miskle, B., Lynch, A., Arndt, S., & Acion, L. (2021). Substance use in pregnancy: Identifying stigma and improving care. *Substance Abuse Rehabilitation, 12*, 105–121. https://doi.org/10.2147/SAR.S319180

Chapter 15
Health Outcomes Among Justice-Involved Mothers

Denae L. Bradley

15.1 Surveillance and Incarceration in the USA

Corrections refers to the incarceration and surveillance of adult and juvenile populations within the USA charged with, or convicted of, committing crimes (United States Department of Justice USDOJ], 1999). The American corrections system consists of institutional corrections facilities that confine individuals who have been convicted of a crime or are awaiting trial, as well as community corrections. Community corrections encompass supervision of individuals convicted of a crime who reside in the community instead of a jail or prison. It is important to note that American correctional agencies with the USA are not uniform. For example, institutional agencies in some states may include community supervision, such as parolee supervision, whereas other states may separate parole from institutional agencies. Nevertheless, this chapter uses the Department of Justice definitions: Institutional corrections refer to prisons and jails, and community corrections refer to probation and parole (USDOJ, 1999).

Since 1971, the prison population has increased by 700%. Scholars argue that Richard Nixon's *War on Drugs*, Bill Clinton's crime bill, and George W. Bush's *War on Terror* created overlapping periods of amplified surveillance, policing, and incarceration of primarily working-class and Black and Brown people (Alexander, 2010; Taylor, 2016). This culmination of events sparked what is commonly referred to as *mass incarceration* (American Civil Liberties Union, 2022).

The War on Drugs is particularly relevant for the incarceration of women because it sparked a change in their involvement with the criminal justice system. In recent

D. L. Bradley (✉)
Robert Wood Johnson Health Policy Research Scholar, Howard University, Hyattsville, MD, USA
e-mail: denae.bradley@bison.howard.edu

© The Author(s), under exclusive license to Springer Nature Switzerland AG 2023   193
B. A. Anderson, L. R. Roberts (eds.), *Maternal Health and American Cultural Values*,
Global Maternal and Child Health, https://doi.org/10.1007/978-3-031-23969-4_15

decades, women's incarceration has grown at twice the rate of men's incarceration (Equal Justice Initiative, 2018). The Sentencing Project, an advocacy group for criminal justice (see https://www.sentencingproject.org/about-us), states that these women are primarily charged with drug or property offenses (Underwood, 2022, May 12). About three-fourths of incarcerated women are of childbearing age (18–44 years), and roughly 70% are mothers and primary caregivers to children under the age of 18. Women of color and poor women are disproportionately affected by mass incarceration. In 2017, 53% of women in prison were women of color. Black women are incarcerated two to three times more than their White counterparts (Bronson & Carson, 2019). These statistics necessitate inquiry into the potential implications of carceral policies and practices on maternal health outcomes.

15.2   Maternal Health Outcomes in Jails and Prisons

The Supreme Court Case, *Estelle v. Gamble*, was a foundational case that established medical care as a constitutional right for incarcerated individuals (Estelle v. Gamble, 1976). Since its enactment, the federal government has outlined policy recommendations on servicing incarcerated individuals, including care for pregnant and postpartum mothers. Many jails and prisons have either in-house or contracted healthcare (Kelsey et al., 2017); however type, quality, and cost vary across carceral settings. Generally, healthcare in jails and prisons is of poor quality, and does not provide adequate care to the high number of persons with comorbidities.

Ample research has shown that incarcerated and formerly incarcerated people experience health disparities and poorer health outcomes than non-incarcerated individuals (Massoglia, 2008a, 2008b; Massoglia & Pridemore, 2015; Schnittker & John, 2007). This research suggests that contact with the criminal justice system contributes to severe healthcare limitations, long-term health problems, elevated stress loads, and racial health disparities. There is, however, limited information on the effects of mass incarceration specifically on maternal health outcomes. American views surrounding incarcerated populations are reflected in the glaring lack of data and disregard for the health of incarcerated mothers.

Many women are pregnant at the time of incarceration. In a study by Pearl & Knittel (2020) around 80% of women surveyed reported being sexually active with men in the months prior to their incarceration, while only 30% reported consistent contraception use. In 2019, Sufrin et al. reported the results of a 12-month prospective study of pregnancy prevalence in 22 state prisons in various geographical regions conducted in 2016–2017. Prior to this study, there had been no systematic collection of prison pregnancy prevalence in American prisons, although the Bureau of Justice Statistics does collect mortality data. This study reported that 1396 pregnant mothers were admitted into these 22 prison sites in the study period, 3.8% of all newly admitted female prisoners. Among the women who gave birth during the study period, there were 753 live births of which 39% were preterm and 30% were cesarean birth. There were 46 miscarriages, 11 abortions, four stillbirths, three newborn deaths, and no maternal deaths. Follow-up studies have shown similar results (Sufrin et al., 2020; Minji, et al., 2021). Sufrin et al. (2020) reported 55,000 pregnant prisoners nationally based upon the 3% admission rate of pregnant women.

15.3   The Framework of Reproductive Justice

The framework of *reproductive justice* helps to contextualize the maternal health crisis in the nation's jails and prisons, including lack of attention to mothers once incarcerated. This contemporary framework was developed by a group of Black American women and assesses the experiences of reproduction (Ross & Solinger, 2017). It is rooted in human rights principles used to justify universal access to community-based resources, such as high-quality healthcare, healthy environments, and sustainable safety nets. Reproductive justice is also a political movement-building framework that critiques prevailing power structures across multiple intersections of oppression. Reproductive justice activists and scholars argue that reproductive experiences must be placed within the community and social contexts in which they occur. Within these experiences, past and current oppressive activities and policies can be examined in relationship to their impact on maternal and reproductive health outcomes. The guiding principles of this framework include: (1) the right to not have a child; (2) the right to have a child; and (3) the right to parent children in safe and healthy environments (Ross & Solinger, 2017).

According to a 2004 Department of Justice report, 54% of incarcerated pregnant women received basic prenatal care. A more recent study reported that all surveyed jail facilities provided a bottom bunk, food supplements, and prenatal vitamins; however, the facilities were less likely to provide liquid supplements or healthy food options for pregnant mothers (Kelsey et al., 2017). The Rebecca Project for Human Rights, a Washington, DC non-profit organization, advocates for policy reform in situations of injustice against women in Africa and the USA. This advocacy includes healthcare policies in jails and prisons (see http://www.rebeccaprojectjustice.org). In 2010, the Rebecca Project found that 38 states had no policies requiring basic prenatal care for incarcerated pregnant women and 41 states did not ensure prenatal diets for incarcerated mothers (Kelsey et al., 2017). Another study reported that almost 30% of the surveyed jails and prisons did not have onsite obstetrical and gynecological care, thus, increasing healthcare costs and delaying treatment for an already vulnerable and growing population (Kelsey et al., 2017).

Incarcerated mothers may lack healthcare and be at high risk for sexual, reproductive, and maternal health problems (Allsworth, 2007; Knittel, 2019; Sufrin, 2017). Pregnancy outcomes in some jails were worse than national trends. For example, although the miscarriage rate in the USA is close to 10%, in states like Arizona, Kansas, and Minnesota, rates of miscarriages in jail were up to 22%. The cesarean birth rate in some states was higher than the national average. Cesarean birth among incarcerated mothers may not always be medically indicated (Sufrin et al., 2019). Earlier studies found high rates of prenatal complications (e.g., preterm labor, gestational diabetes, and hypertension) in the prison population (Cordero et al., 1992; Lin, 1997). Incarcerated mothers were significantly more likely to have chronic health problems that impact pregnancy outcomes compared to free-living mothers. Many of these medical problems, like epilepsy, cardiac or renal disease, and diabetes, increase the risk of adverse maternal health outcomes (Knight & Plugge, 2005). However, some studies report similar rates of adverse maternal health outcomes among low-income, marginalized mothers and incarcerated mothers (Egley et al., 1992; Fogel, 1993). It is important to note that Black women, poor women, and rural women face similar health disparities and are often overrepresented in the criminal legal system. The severity of these disparities is generally exacerbated once these women are incarcerated (Knittel, 2019).

Few scholars study the maternal and reproductive health experiences of incarcerated women. Obstetrician-gynecologist, medical anthropologist, and researcher Dr. Carolyn Sufrin is one such scholar. Dr. Sufrin is an associate professor at John Hopkins University School of Medicine. I (DB) interviewed her, asking her to explain how American cultural values around motherhood are related to incarcerated women's access to maternal and reproductive healthcare. Her response, in her words, in the interview in Box 15.1 calls attention to the reproductive injustices that stratify Black and poor women based on their assumed criminality and lack of ability to parent.

Box 15.1 Interview with Carolyn Sufrin, MD, PhD, Author of Jailcare: Finding the Safety Net for Women Behind Bars

When it comes to the healthcare that [incarcerated mothers or pregnant women] do or do not receive while they're in custody, it's not only about that baseline…"What does an incarcerated person deserve?" "Do they deserve better healthcare?" as some of my research informants who are correctional officers [have asked].

What you get on top of that is the value or devaluation of their fitness as mothers and as parents and that's linked to an anthropological concept we call *stratified reproduction* - the notion that some people's reproduction and procreative capacities and abilities to mother and to parent are supported and encouraged and valued in society while other people's reproduction, procreation, and parenting are actively suppressed and devalued.

We have to understand it is so fundamentally situated in our country's history of enslavement and of White supremacy, and what kinds of motherhood have been held up as the example of the ideal to achieve and which kinds of motherhood have been vilified and criminalized. There is a lengthy answer to that question, and there is also a short answer, which is that the idealized version of motherhood is White, middle, and upper class, and grounded in composition of nuclear family.

Black motherhood is very systematically devalued and actively suppressed, and there is a long legacy and historical iterations of this differential evaluation. We see it manifested very clearly in incarcerated mothers who are disproportionately Black and who, even when they are in the community, are affected by systems, such as the so-called child welfare system or what I more aptly called a family regulation system. That, even when they're not incarcerated, their motherhood is so highly regulated and devalued, and we see that take that same form as being incarcerated.

When I asked Dr. Sufrin about barriers to being self-reliant for previously incarcerated mothers, her response initiated a discussion on the broader structures that make it impossible for them to parent and have healthy pregnancies. She also discussed the potential drawbacks of using self-reliance as a measure of success, particularly for those in carceral environments with a severely limited ability to make choices.

(Personal communication, Carolyn Sufrin, January 12, 2022)

Dr. Sufrin's response captures one of the critical premises of this chapter: A person's access to healthcare and ability to parent is necessarily tethered to their social position and alliance with American cultural values, such as self-reliance. The following sections will examine the American cultural value of self-reliance in relation to policies and practices for incarcerated pregnant mothers.

15.4 Self-Reliance: An American Cultural Value

Cultural values influence decision-making and resource distribution with implications for health inequities and adverse social determinants of health (SDoH). Disadvantaged groups may be deprived of resources, thus negatively impacting their health (Williams, 2003). The cultural value of self-reliance expects responsibility without undue dependence upon others. Lack of self-reliance is strongly condemned within American culture. For example, individuals who self-medicate during pregnancy, resulting in adverse maternal and infant outcomes, may be described as lacking self-reliance. Pregnant mothers who use drugs may tell a different story. Self-medicating may help them cope with the realities of poverty and structural inequalities without the assistance of others. Both scenarios express the cultural value of self-reliance. How does one become self-reliant in a society that unequally distributes and denies resources?

15.4.1 The Myth of Self-Reliance

Sociologists Stephen McNamee and Robert Miller (2004) argue that America's distribution of income is highly skewed, which refutes "any reasonable distribution of merit" (p. 3). No one lives an entirely self-reliant life. While many Americans praise entrepreneurs as self-made individuals, such individuals did not independently create the economy nor the infrastructure that makes their endeavors possible. Complex networks are necessary to achieve success. McNamee and Miller purport that there is a "gap between how people think the system works and how the system actually works," which they refer to as the *meritocracy myth* (2004:1). They identify some non-merit factors, such as inheritance and discrimination, that can promote or create barriers to social mobility. For example, those born with higher class placement and/or an inheritance start life with social advantages compared to those who grew up poor. On the other hand, merit comes second to coping with cumulative life events including health disparities, cumulative stress, and inequality—the SDoH as described in *Healthy People* 2030 (Healthy People, 2030).

Self-reliance is a myth, not a reality. Mary Midgley, a moral philosopher, claims that myths "…are imaginative patterns, networks of powerful symbols that suggest particular ways of interpreting the world. They shape its meaning" (2004, p. 2). Myths also justify our existence. William Doty, a scholar of religion, argues that myths provide a rationale for the "…many issues of what a culture considers to be appropriate behaviors and models of selfhood, as well as models of social and political ways of existing" (Midgley, 2004, p. 2). The myth of self-reliance justifies rising inequality in America, including mass incarceration and poor maternal health outcomes (McNamee & Miller, 2004).

15.4.2   Criminalizing Non-Adherence to Self-Reliance

Cultural values explain why certain groups are positively viewed while others are ostracized and criminalized (Foucault, 1995; Nicholson-Crotty, 2004; Schneider et al., 2014; Schnittker & John, 2007). No studies were located that specifically investigated how cultural values are expressed in the decision-making processes affecting mothers in corrections. However, social constructions that characterize the *haves* and *have-nots* have important implications for examining the potential impact of cultural values on carceral healthcare policies, programs, and practices (Williams, 2003).

15.4.2.1   Exemplar: Self-Reliance and Healthcare

In America's growing carceral state, increased criminalization has become the response to growing social inequalities and unequal distribution of resources, including access to healthcare (Alexander, 2010; Bach, 2014; Phelan & Link, 2015; Ritchie, 2017; Wilson & O'Brien, 2016). The social determinants of poverty and structural inequalities assure that mothers in the criminal justice system have difficulty accessing the resources needed to maintain good health for themselves and their children. Those who lack self-reliance skills may be stigmatized for violating this cultural value but may not be given the necessary resources—a commentary on the failing public health safety net (Sufrin, 2017).

15.4.2.2   Exemplar: Self-Reliance and Substance Abuse

The American legal system criminalizes maternal substance abuse with punitive child abuse or neglect policies. Many state drug policies encourage healthcare providers to alert the criminal justice system if a pregnant woman reports or is suspected of drug use (Ritchie, 2017). Yet, emerging research suggests that states with punitive or reporting policies do not demonstrate decreased substance abuse and have an increased likelihood of poor infant health outcomes, such as neonatal abstinence syndrome (NAS) (Faherty et al., 2019). State-level policymakers may use judgments based upon the cultural value of self-reliance in their decisions. The 1980 Medical University of South Carolina task force is an example of how the cultural value of self-reliance influences policies that criminalize minoritized communities. This university developed a joint-task force with the Charleston police department, local prosecutors, and healthcare providers to *protect the fetuses* of *low-income women seeking prenatal care who tested positive for cocaine.* The task force argued that a fetus is a *living person* and deserves protection under state law. According to court documents, they claimed that drug-addicted pregnant women could be guilty of distributing illicit drugs to minors. Based upon a 1989 task force report, over 200 women have tested positive for drug use without consenting to a drug test. While the policy offered education and referrals to drug treatment programs, the task force threatened more punitive interventions. An estimated 40 mothers were arrested, and nearly all of them were Black (Legal Information Institute, 2001; Ferguson v. Charleston, 2001). In this example, state agents and healthcare officials joined forces to punish and incarcerate minority pregnant women who did not demonstrate self-reliance in drug counseling. This case, heard in the Supreme Court, sent a message about lack of compliance with a cultural value. It also reinforced stereotypes about Black mothers and their ability to parent their children (Roberts, 2017; Ross & Solinger, 2017).

15.4.2.3   Exemplar: Self-Reliance and Reproductive Violence in Prison

The cultural value of self-reliance can influence decisions within the carceral healthcare system.

Numerous studies recount obstetrical violence by correctional officers, healthcare providers, and an ill-equipped carceral healthcare system (Cross, 2019; Kelsey et al., 2017; Knittel, 2019; Paltrow & Flavin, 2013; Sufrin, 2017). For example, Erika Cohn, in her stunning and disturbing film, *Belly of the Beast,* documents the state-sanctioned forced sterilizations of women housed in California prisons (Cohn, 2020, 0:81). The Center for Investigative Reporting reports that roughly 148 pregnant incarcerated women underwent tubal ligations between 2006 and 2010 after giving birth in prison. Most of these women, both Black and Latinx, were targeted by correctional staff because they were deemed at risk for recidivism. Narratives from incarcerated women detail the coercive methods doctors used to get them to agree to sterilization. Some women were pushed to sign paperwork that they did not understand or were asked to sign medical forms while sedated and shackled to surgical tables (Johnson, 2013, July 7). Some were coerced into signing sterilization consent forms (Roth & Ainsworth, 2015). Stories from carceral healthcare providers suggest their actions were influenced by growing concerns about marginalized women depending on welfare programs instead of being self-sufficient. This example is a glaring connection to the historical control of minority and low-income women's reproductive capacity with implications for their maternal health outcomes (Cohn, 2020, 0:81).

15.4.3 Policies and Programs to Support Self-Reliance

In response to the growing number of mothers in corrections, the criminal justice system has implemented some policies and programs to support their health and parenting. These programs provide access to doula services, prenatal supplements and diets, modifications in living and work standards, breastfeeding support, and other services that support parenting and positive maternal health outcomes (Pendleton et al., 2020). For example, the Minnesota Prison Doula Project, a partnership of the community, the university, and the corrections division, provides programming to support pregnant incarcerated women (Shlafer et al., 2015). This project offers weekly parenting classes and one-on-one doula support in response to incarcerated mothers' concerns about prenatal development, the birth process, and parenting. A doula is a trained individual who provides emotional and physical support and resources to pregnant people and their families. Although they do not have healthcare training, they are trained in supporting labor, childbirth, and the postpartum period. Doula support is significant for incarcerated mothers because many prisons do not allow family members into birthing sites (Pendleton et al., 2020). Programs like this may support self-reliance among incarcerated mothers, although overall, there is little empirical evidence that policies and programs actually foster self-reliance (Pendleton et al., 2020; Sufrin, 2017).

15.5 Summary

This chapter argues that self-reliance, a key American cultural value, influences policies and decisions inside and outside the carceral setting. Mothers who lack resources and self-reliance while dealing with structural inequalities are often penalized, increasing their risk for poor maternal health outcomes. SDoH, including inadequate and unstable housing, gender-based violence, stigma, racism, and limited access to healthy foods and quality healthcare, have important implications for the health and well-being of incarcerated mothers. They also establish why there is much overlap between those at risk of being incarcerated and those more likely to experience poor maternal health outcomes.

At the community level, incarceration disproportionately impacts some communities more than others. High rates of mass incarceration burden Black and Brown people and those in poverty, stripping valuable human and social capital from their communities and contributing to poor maternal health outcomes. This is particularly important for future research on the links of structural racism, cultural values, and maternal health.

Healthy People 2030 (Healthy People, 2030) identifies incarceration as an adverse SDoH. One of the goals is to reduce the proportion of children with a mother in corrections; however, current policies that criminalize the inability to be self-reliant disproportionately increase the proportion of minority and low-income children who have a mother who has served time in jail. Research shows that incarcerated mothers with a history of substance use are more likely to disengage from the healthcare system once released from jail or prison (Faherty et al., 2019). These same women also struggle to parent their children and raise their families with dignity. This is partly because laws terminating parental rights disproportionately impact poor, minority, and justice-involved families. Those policymakers who punish people for lacking self-reliance blame these mothers. Justice-involved mothers are caught in the web of a failed safety net.

References

Alexander, M. (2010). *The new Jim crow: Mass incarceration in the age of colorblindness.* New Press.

Allsworth, J., Clarke, J., Jeffrey, P., Hebert, M., Cooper, A., & Boardman, L. (2007). The influence of stress on the menstrual cycle among newly incarcerated women. *Women's Health Issues, 17,* 202–209. https://doi.org/10.1016/j.whi.2007.02.002

American Civil Liberties Union. (2022). *Mass incarceration.* ACLU. https://www.aclu.org/issues/smart-justice/mass-incarceration

Bach, W. (2014). The hyperregulatory state: Women, race, poverty, and support. *Yale Journal of Law and Feminism, 25*(2).

Bronson, J. & Carson, A. (2019, April). Prisoners in 2017. Bureau of Justices Statistics, 252156. 1–43. https://bjs.ojp.gov/content/pub/pdf

Cross, J. (2019). Incarcerating pregnant and parenting women, the new witch hunt: A policy analysis. *Maternal and Child Health Journal, 23,* 431–434. https://doi.org/10.1007/s10995-019-02739-y

Cohn, E. (Director). (2020). Belly of the Beast [Documentary Film], *Idle Wild Films.* https://www.bellyofthebeastfilm.com

Cordero, L., Hines, S., Shibley, K. A., & Landon, M. B. (1992). Perinatal outcomes for women in prison. *Journal of Perinatology, 12*(3), 205–209.

Egley, C. C., Miller, D. E., Granados, J. L., & Ingram-Fogel, C. (1992). Outcome of pregnancy during imprisonment. *Journal of Reproductive Medicine, 37*(2), 131–134.

Equal Justice Initiative. (2018). *Incarceration of women is growing twice as fast as that of men. Equal Justice Initiative.* https://eji.org/news/female-incarceration-growing-twice-as-fast-as-male-incarceration/

Estelle v. Gamble, 429 U.S. 97 (1976).

Faherty, L., Kranz, A. M., Russell-Fritch, J., Patrick, S. W., Cantor, J., & Stein, B. D. (2019). Association of punitive and reporting state policies related to substance use in pregnancy with rates of neonatal abstinence syndrome. *JAMA Network Open, 2*(11), e1914078. https://doi.org/10.1001/jamanetworkopen.2019.14078

Fogel, C. I. (1993). Pregnant inmates risk factors and pregnancy outcomes. *Journal of Obstetric, Gynecologic & Neonatal Nursing, 22*(1), 33–39. https://doi.org/10.1111/j.1552-6909.1993.tb01780.x

Foucault, M. (1995). *Discipline and punish: The birth of the prison.* Vintage Books.

Ferguson v. Charleston, 532 U.S. 67 (2001).

Healthy People. (2030). U.S. Department of Health and Human Services, Office of Disease Prevention and Health Promotion. https://health.gov/healthypeople/objectives-and-data/social-determinants-health

Johnson, C. (2013, July 7). Female inmates sterilized in California prisons without approval. *The Center for Investigative Reporting.* https://revealnews.org/article/dremale-inmates-sterilized-in-california-prisons-without-approval

Kelsey, C. M., Medel, N., Mullins, C., Dallaire, D., & Forestell, C. (2017). An examination of care practices of pregnant women incarcerated in jail facilities in the United States. *Maternal and Child Health Journal, 21*(6), 1260–1266. https://doi.org/10.1007/s10995-016-2224-5

Knight, M., & Plugge, E. (2005). Risk factors for adverse perinatal outcomes in imprisoned pregnant women: A systematic review. *BMC Public Health, 5*(1), 111.

Knittel, A. (2019). Resolving health disparities for women involved in the criminal justice system. *North Carolina Medical Journal, 80*(6), 363–366. https://doi.org/10.18043/ncm.80.6.363

Legal Information Institute (2001). Ferguson v. Charleston. *Cornell Law School.* https://www.law.cornell.edu/supct/html/99-936.ZO,html

Lin, C. (1997). *Patterns of care and outcomes for pregnant inmates and their infants in Texas state prisons: Epidemiologic and ethnographic analyses. Unpublished doctoral dissertation.* University of Texas School of Public Health, ProQuest – Dissertation (9809602).

Massoglia, M. (2008a). Incarceration, health, and racial disparities in health. *Law & Society Review, 42*(2), 275–306.

Massoglia, M. (2008b). Incarceration as exposure: The prison, infectious disease, and other stress-related illnesses. *Journal of Health and Social Behavior, 49*(1), 56–71.

Massoglia, M., & Pridemore, W. (2015). Incarceration and health. *Annual Review of Sociology, 41*, 291–310.

McNamee, S. J., & Miller, R. K. (2004). *The meritocracy myth. Sociation Today, 2*(1), 1–13.

Midgley, M. (2004). *The myths we live by.* Routledge.

Minji, K., Sufrin, C., Nowotny, K., Beal, L., & Jiménez, M. (2021, Aug). Pregnancy prevalence and outcomes in 3 United States juvenile residential systems. *Journal of Pediatric & Adolescent Gynecology, 34*(4), 546–551. https://doi.org/10.1016/j.jpag.2021.01.005

Nicholson-Crotty, J., & Nicholson-Crotty, S. (2004). Social construction and policy implementation: Inmate health as a public health issue. *Social Science Quarterly, 85*(2), 240–257.

Paltrow, L., & Flavin, J. (2013). Arrests of and forced interventions on pregnant women in the United States, 1973–2005: Implications for women's legal status and public health. *Journal of Health Politics Policy Law, 38*(2), 299–343. https://doi.org/10.1215/03616878-1966324

Pearl, M., & Knittel, A. (2020). Contraception need and available services among incarcerated women in the United States: A systematic review. *Contraception and Reproductive Medicine, 5*, 2020. https://doi.org/10.1186/s40834-020-00105-w

Pendleton, V., Saunders, J., & Shlafer, R. (2020). Corrections officers' knowledge and perspectives of maternal and child health policies and programs for pregnant women in prison. *Health and Justice, 8*(1), 1. https://doi.org/10.1186/s40352-019-0102-0

Phelan, J. C., & Link, B. G. (2015). Is racism a fundamental cause of inequalities in health? *Annual Review of Sociology, 41*, 311–330. https://doi.org/10.1146/annurev-soc-073014-112305

Ritchie, A. (2017). *Invisible no more: Police violence against black women and women of color.* Beacon Press.

Roberts, D. E. (2017). *Killing the black body: Race, reproduction, and the meaning of liberty.* Vintage Books.

Ross, L., & Solinger, R. (2017). *Reproductive justice: An introduction.* University of California Press.

Roth, R., & Ainsworth, S. (2015). 'If they hand you a paper, you sign it': A call to end the sterilization of women in prison. *Hastings Women's Law Journal, 26*(1), 7–50.

Schneider, A., Ingram, H., & DeLeon, P. (2014). Democratic policy design: Social construction of target populations. In P. Sabatier & C. Weible (Eds.), *Theories of the policy process* (3rd ed., pp. 105–150). Westview Press.

Schnittker, J., & John, A. (2007). Enduring stigma: The long-term effects of incarceration on health. *Journal of Health and Social Behavior, 48*(2), 115–130. https://doi.org/10.1177/002214650704800202

Shlafer, R. J., Gerrity, E., & Duwe, G. (2015). Pregnancy and parenting support for incarcerated women: Lessons learned_progress in community health partnerships : Research, education, and action. *Progress in Community Health Partnerships, 9*(3), 371–378. https://doi.org/10.1353/cpr.2015.0061

Sufrin, C. (2017). *Jailcare: Finding the safety net for women behind bars.* University of California Press.

Sufrin, C., Beal, L., Clarke, J., Jones, R., & Mosher, W. (2019). Pregnancy outcomes in US prisons, 2016-2017. *American Journal of Public Health, 109*, 799–805. https://doi.org/10.2105/AJPH.2019.305006

Sufrin, C., Jones, R., Mosher, W., & Beal, L. (2020). Pregnancy prevalence and outcomes in U.S. jails. *Obstetrics & Gynecology, 135*(5), 1177–1183. https://doi.org/10.1097/AOG.0000000000003834

Taylor, K. Y. (2016). *From #BlackLivesMatter to black liberation.* Haymarket Books.

Underwood, W. (2022, May 12). Incarcerated women and girls. The Sentencing Project. https://www.sentencingproject.org/publications/incarcerated-women-and-girls/.

United States Department of Justice. (1999). New directions from the field: Victims' rights and services for the 21st century. Office of Justice Programs & Office for Victims of Crime. https:www.ncjrs,gov/ovc_archives/directions/pdftxt.pdf.

Williams, L. (2003). *The constraint of race: Legacies of white skin privilege in America.* Penn State University Press.

Willison, J., & O'Brien, P. (2016). A feminist call for transforming the criminal justice system. *Affilia, 32*(1), 37–49. https://doi.org/10.1177/0886109916658080

Part V
Reflections in the Cultural Mirror

Chapter 16
Conclusions

Lisa R. Roberts and Barbara A. Anderson

16.1 Reflections on History, Values, and Decisions

Maternal health in the USA has historically lagged behind other high-resource nations, and continues to do so currently, despite high healthcare expenditures and numerous targeted efforts to improve maternal health metrics. Hampering progress is the focus on the social determinants of health (SDoH) as the endpoint in understanding the high rates of maternal mortality and morbidity, near misses, and poor childbearing outcomes. SDoH contribute to an understanding of conditions influencing maternal health and drive decisions at all levels on maternal healthcare programming. These SDoH answer key questions of *who, what, when, where,* and *how much* social and environmental conditions contribute to adverse maternal health outcomes. They define maternal populations at high risk. What they do not explain is *why* these disparities persist, even as other high-resource nations have embarked upon programming at all economic levels to protect the health of mothers with demonstrated better outcomes.

In this book, we offer a critical analysis of the question *why* within one perspective—the American history and cultural values. In order to *intentionalize* decisions that drive positive outcomes and evaluate decisions with poor maternal health outcomes, we have explored five predominant American cultural values (personal control; individualism; action-orientation; practicality; and self-reliance) and their influence on decisions about maternal health. How motherhood has been viewed historically and how it has evolved over time are important in understanding the experiences of motherhood in the USA. Life course theory provides a framework

L. R. Roberts (✉)
Loma Linda University, Loma Linda, CA, USA

B. A. Anderson
Frontier Nursing University, Versailles, KY, USA

© The Author(s), under exclusive license to Springer Nature Switzerland AG 2023
B. A. Anderson, L. R. Roberts (eds.), *Maternal Health and American Cultural Values*,
Global Maternal and Child Health, https://doi.org/10.1007/978-3-031-23969-4_16

for placing mothers' experiences within American cultural values, going beyond data metrics, to describe personal control, self-reliance, and individualism. Building a family or choosing not to become a mother are grounded in values of action-orientation and practicality.

Maternal health is influenced by mental and physical health status, personal experiences in the family and community, minority and/or immigrant status, the impact of othering, media messaging, health services, and the justice system, among others. In order to address the question of *why* the USA has poor health outcomes among many mothers, looking into the cultural mirror can provide some insights. The varied path to motherhood in America reflects our varied population. Expectations of family structure and the motherhood mandate are deeply rooted in the USA, and the cultural values of practicality and action-orientation further influence women's experiences of infertility, distress or ambivalence about motherhood, and decision-making around assisted reproduction. Negative birth experiences and expectations of respectful maternity care both influence and reflect the value placed on motherhood in America.

Maternal mental health, particularly in the postpartum period, is directly affected by experiences of systemic discrimination, and at the same time, expectations related to the cultural value of personal control. Systemic discrimination, which persists in the context of historical and cultural influences, is evident in the SDoH domain of social and community context. Personal control is a cultural value that may increase the risk of postpartum mental health issues, as loss of personal control is inherent to the childbearing process, yet highly stigmatized. Thus, mothers are often caught in the middle, navigating the tensions of opposing forces. Their decision-making occurs at the individual level, in the context of family and community, and within the influences of American society at large. Mothers living in the military community experience unique circumstances often beyond individual control. Yet practicality and self-reliance are expected and highly valued. Immigrant and refugee mothers, as well as those at the USA-Mexico border, reflect skills and stresses with living out the values of person control. Those who are marginalized and discriminated against display both resilience and the weathering demanded by these efforts. The individualism and autonomy of American mothers are both lauded and thwarted by conflicting cultural messages and rhetoric.

While healthcare ethics support maternal autonomy, social polarization on cultural values influence women's choices about pregnancy timing, continuation, and birth planning. Autonomy also does not play out equally for all mothers—women of lower socioeconomic status often bearing the brunt of political decision-making and policy implementation more than women of higher socioeconomic status. Additionally, while autonomy may be viewed differently among various groups, particularly when collectivism is emphasized over individualism, supporting motherhood with accurate information, product availability, and access to services is essential. Recent examples from the COVID-19 pandemic show the impact of decisions and cultural values on the public health safety net of the USA. While controlling COVID-19 was prioritized, anti-science sentiments fueled polarization and maternal health services were interrupted. Reflected in the SDoH, available and affordable child care, interpersonal violence, neighborhood security, human traf-ficking, access to weapons, criminalization of addictions, and justice in incarcera-tion are all issues influenced by cultural values and affecting maternal health outcomes.

Outside of the military, decisions about management of an aging infrastructure and porous safety net affect survival services and population health. The impact on maternal health is far more evident in poor communities and stands in stark contrast to other high-resource nations where greater political unity exists. Some American mothers struggle in communities where SDoH significantly influence maternal out-comes as safe water, insecure and substandard housing, crime, and food deserts threaten health. Stronger maternal health policies are needed to benefit every mother. Meanwhile, examples of concerned citizens who have taken practical action to help mitigate food deserts, contaminated water, poor housing, and air pollution reflect the cultural values of action-orientation and practicality.

Immigrant, refugee, and undocumented mothers present an interesting paradoxi-cal effect of adverse SDoH and the American cultural value of personal control as they navigate motherhood in their new homeland. These mothers often find it diffi-cult to maintain healthy behaviors when faced with an unfamiliar environment fraught with challenges such as accessing healthcare, food deserts, health literacy, and safety. Their initial resilience and prior personal control may be temporarily daunted as they adjust. Some in the subsequent generations continue to struggle, ultimately reflecting the struggles of the general American population. *Why* superior maternal health outcomes are not maintained among immigrant populations is trou-bling, perhaps reflecting the historical impact of *othering* and perceptions and myths about who is fit for motherhood.

Systemic racism, discrimination, and SDoH that are beyond the personal control of the mothers affected lead to poor maternal health outcomes and reflect the gen-eral valuing of White middle-class motherhood in the USA. *Othering* and judgment regarding fitness for motherhood detrimentally affect mothers physiologically and psychologically, as well as contributing to suboptimal healthcare access and quality, ultimately vulnerability. *Othered* women have demonstrated resilience through their lived experiences outside of majority norms, which reflect the American cultural value of personal control, yet society lacks a willingness to accept and support these mothers equitably. This lack of acceptance and the resulting inequities are high-lighted in the daily headlines across the USA.

Birth practices are influenced by personal experience as well as historical and cultural values. Choices regarding the timing and/or continuation of pregnancy are hotly debated as policy decision-making is currently in flux, disrupting the once stable context of *Roe v. Wade* (Roe v. Wade, 1973). The restriction on availability of abortion, as well as the severe criminalization of abortion varies from state to state. While some states have chosen to be safe harbors to protect maternal autonomy, as of this writing, at least one state had legislation under consideration to make abor-tion punishable by death (LaMarco, 2022; Winter et al., 2022). As these issues con-tinue to develop in the courts, the impact on maternal health is dubious. Public opinion and media messaging, inherently linked, influence the national conversation on these issues.

Media messaging plays a significant role in American motherhood. Not only does media reflect cultural values, it also engenders current views of the role of motherhood, who is fit to be a mother, and who is subject to poor maternal health outcomes. Media messaging, with accurate information, misinformation, and disinformation, contributes to decisions that drive policy implementation. Healthcare providers see the dual effects of policy and adverse SDoH affecting mothers. Poverty, limited education and health literacy, racism, adverse childhood events, mental illness, substance abuse, interaction with the judicial system, and intimate partner violence are associated with predictable adverse effects on maternal health. Healthcare providers are expected to demonstrate action-orientation in decision-making, playing an important role in both lived experiences and maternal health outcomes.

With mass incarceration, disproportionally affects justice-involved mothers who are Black, Brown, or in poverty. Healthcare providers must balance policy implementation and providing evidence-based care while caring for justice-involved mothers. Self-reliance is often an unrealistic cultural value within the contexts of these women's lives both before and after justice involvement. Similarly, substance abuse is often perceived as evidence of lack of self-reliance. Mothers who use substances are often blamed for having the problem and expected to "pull themselves up by the bootstraps" to resolve the problem. These mothers are at risk for justice involvement, putting them at additional risk for poor maternal health outcomes. The pervasive cultural polarization around these issues influences policy changes and implementation.

Additional high-risk contexts include intimate partner violence, lack of neighborhood security, access to weapons, and human trafficking. These adverse SDoH decrease maternal autonomy and safety. Reflecting the American cultural value of individualism, mothers are often expected to achieve their goals even with obstacles beyond their control. In contrast, individualism balanced by collaboration and consideration for others (e.g., public health) reflects the best possible strengths of the nation and can influence policy decision-making and positively affect maternal safety and autonomy.

16.2   Advancing Maternal Health in America: The Path Forward

Historically, American cultural values have had deep influence on the decisions made in this nation. They currently ground our decision-making processes at all levels. Examination of how these cultural values impact outcomes compels us to take a hard look beyond the obvious. It prods us to go beyond the social determinants that are easily explanatory for poor maternal health outcomes. It helps us to explore how our values influence the decisions that affect the lives of our mothers. It goes beyond the usual diagnostic metrics—*who, what, when, where,* and *how much* to ask the question **why**. Why do we do what we do? Why do we make decisions that allow poor outcomes? Why are we, an affluent nation, an outlier with such high maternal mortality and morbidity?

Looking through the cultural mirror allows us to reflect, to shine a light on the blemishes but also on the inherent beauty of our values. Ida B. Wells-Barrett, Black leader in the post-Civil War reconstruction period, noted that it takes courage to shine this light (see https://www.goodreads.com/author/quotes/102474.Ida_B_Wells_Barnett). American writer James Thurber reflected, "It is better to know some of the questions than all of the answers," (Thurber, 1990, p. 28).

We know some, not all of the answers, about poor maternal health outcomes and about the social determinants that erode health—poverty, food insecurity, violence, and racism. Do we have the courage to ask the last question? Why do we do what we do? Examining decision-making within the framework of American cultural values can help to address this question. It can provide guidance in building strength and facing weakness. It can provide a healthier path forward for American mothers.

References

LaMarco, N. (2022). States are pursuing "Safe Harbor" laws: How will they impact healthcare? Ask. https://www.ask.com/news/state-safe-harbor-laws-healthcare

Roe v. Wade, 410 U.S. 113 (1973).

Thurber, J. (1990). *Fables for our time and famous poems illustrated* (p. 28). Harper Perennial.

Winter, E., Datil, A., & Bragg, M. (2022, July 26). Yes, a bill punishing abortion with death was introduced in North Carolina. Verify. https://www.verifythis.com/article/news/verify/government-verify/north-carolina-abortion-death-penalty-bill-introduced-2021-and-stalled/536-9506beb1-ec76-4c4e-abbe-778c45fedee3

Index

© The Editor(s) (if applicable) and The Author(s), under exclusive license to Springer Nature Switzerland AG 2023
B. A. Anderson, L. R. Roberts (eds.), *Maternal Health and American Cultural Values*, Global Maternal and Child Health, https://doi.org/10.1007/978-3-031-23969-4

Printed in the United States
by Baker & Taylor Publisher Services